HUMAN FACTORS
in the
MARITIME DOMAIN

HUMAN FACTORS
in the
MARITIME DOMAIN

Michelle Rita Grech
Tim John Horberry
Thomas Koester

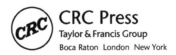

CRC Press
Taylor & Francis Group
Boca Raton London New York

CRC Press is an imprint of the
Taylor & Francis Group, an **informa** business

CRC Press
Taylor & Francis Group
6000 Broken Sound Parkway NW, Suite 300
Boca Raton, FL 33487-2742

First issued in paperback 2019

ISBN-13: 978-1-4200-4341-9 (hbk)
ISBN-13: 978-0-367-37648-2 (pbk)

Library of Congress Cataloging-in-Publication Data

Grech, Michelle.
   Human factors in the maritime domain / Michelle Grech, Tim Horberry, Thomas Koester.
      p. cm.
   Includes bibliographical references and index.
   ISBN 978-1-4200-4341-9 (alk. paper)
   1. Navigation--Safety measures. 2. Collisions at sea. 3. Human-machine systems. I. Horberry, Tim. II. Koester, Thomas. III. Title.

VK371.G73 2008
363.12'31--dc22   2007040539

Visit the Taylor & Francis Web site at
http://www.taylorandfrancis.com

and the CRC Press Web site at
http://www.crcpress.com

Contents

Preface

Human factors is a scientific, theoretical, and applied discipline dealing with psychological, physical, and organizational aspects of the interaction between humans and systems (e.g., technology)—primarily in occupational contexts. The field largely developed based on a realization that the systematic consideration of the human element can make a major contribution in safety-critical domains.

The main purpose of this book is to provide the reader with a much needed overview of human factors within the maritime domain. It is our intention that the book will be useful and interesting for professionals in the field, researchers, and lay readers alike. This book is primarily intended for a maritime audience, which includes seafarers, maritime administrations, classification societies, surveyors, maritime accident investigators, maritime training and research institutes, students, and lecturers alike. We hope that this book will also interest other readers including ship designers, ship managers and operators, and anyone interested in transport safety and human factors. Human factors knowledge is not a prerequisite for reading this book, although some familiarity with the area would certainly be advantageous.

But why is this book necessary? There is a growing realization within the maritime community that consideration of human factors issues is vital. Similar to other transportation domains, human performance problems constitute a significant threat to system safety, making the study of human factors an important field for improving safety at sea. Contrary to the aviation domain, however, very little research and documentation has been published on human factors in the maritime domain. In addition, the piecemeal fashion in which human factors research has been conducted in this domain makes information retrieval available only via research journals or conference papers. We believe that this book is timely because, to date, there is no publication available that presents maritime human factors knowledge and research from a multidisciplinary perspective and combines it into one readable volume. Therefore, such a book seems long overdue in the current market.

The approach taken in the book is holistic, based on a model of the sociotechnical system of work in the maritime domain. The ingredients in this system model include humans (e.g., individual crewmembers, human physiology, psychological limitations, etc.), groups (e.g., crew, communication, team skills, etc.), technology (e.g., ship, instruments, equipment, tools, etc.), work practices (e.g., informal rules, customs, etc.), organizations (e.g., management, procedures, policies, etc.), society and culture (e.g., sociopolitical environment, etc.), and the physical environment (e.g., light, noise, vibration, workspace, etc.).

The relevance of human factors in the maritime domain is obvious when accidents and incidents occur. The human element is a widely recognized frontline origin of mistakes, failures, wrong decisions, poor communication, and so forth. Some very early approaches had a tendency to focus on the individual human as the "error producer." Recent findings have shown that it is only possible to get a full understanding of the mechanisms in accidents and incidents if the human element is viewed as part of a larger system, which includes the technology, organization, practice, and work environment. Accidents and incidents occur when there is a breakdown in the sociotechnical system. This breakdown could be related to, or caused by, for example, poor design of equipment (human–technology) or inconsistencies between work practice and written procedures (work practice–organization). Hence, the cause of the incident or accident is not found in the individual but in the system as a whole. Therefore, when looking for the underlying cause, human error is not the source of the accident, but is the starting point.

The authors acknowledge that the topic of human factors is vast and covers a broad area. This book therefore integrates relevant human factors knowledge in the maritime domain into one single volume. This book starts by putting the topic into an historical and theoretical context, and then moves on to more specific and detailed topics relevant to the maritime domain. It brings together human factors information available from within this and other domains in order to provide vital background information necessary for acquiring a core knowledge base of human factors within the maritime domain. It emphatically presents a theoretical and scientific perspective in maritime human factors. As much as possible we have also given real examples and case studies in the topics outlined, which will provide readers with a more practical outlook. We feel that this allows the reader to see the concrete significance of the material presented while making the text rigorous, useful, and enjoyable.

Given the increasing importance of the human element in maritime operations, it is anticipated that this book will provide the much needed impetus to encourage growth in theoretical and practical research in the area of human factors within the maritime domain. This includes research in new maritime technology such as "enhanced navigation" and consideration of the effects of increased automation in the engine room.

The three authors bring to the book a range of diverse backgrounds in the general area; this has included working as maritime surveyor, transport consultant, human factors lecturer, and mechanical engineer. They have undertaken maritime research in Denmark, Australia, Malta, and the United Kingdom. In addition, they have published several other human factors books in related topics. This combination of human factors knowledge, maritime wisdom, and substantial publication experience will, we hope, produce a book that is effective, practical, and enjoyable.

Acknowledgments

The authors are extremely indebted and grateful to a number of people who in one way or another contributed to the completion of this book. We wish to acknowledge specifically the invaluable help provided by our colleague Steve Boyd from the Defence Science and Technology Organisation (DSTO) for the hours spent proofreading the whole manuscript, making many valuable suggestions for alterations, and patiently going through it with the authors. We are also indebted to Kevin Gaylor and Janis Cocking also from the DSTO who wholeheartedly supported this project from day one. Kevin Gaylor's enthusiasm and encouragement when we first mentioned this project was a real source of inspiration and this continued through completion of the manuscript. Special mention must be made of a very good friend, Carmelo Vassallo, coordinator of the Mediterranean Maritime History Network (MMHN), who was involved in the project at the beginning, directing us to the appropriate resources and material utilized in the work. We also acknowledge the support of Paul Elischer and Jim Brown of the DSTO. Special thanks go to our editor at CRC Press, Cindy Carelli, for her continuous patience and understating during the writing up process.

Without the encouragement and support from these people this book would never have been possible.

Finally we extend our warmest thanks to our families, in particular Andre, Patricie, and Lisbeth for putting up with us, and for just being there!

The Authors

Michelle Rita Grech. Michelle works for the Maritime Platforms Division within the Defence Science and Technology Organisation (DSTO) in Australia. Her current work involves maritime-focused research on human systems integration and human factors. She joined DSTO after completing her Ph.D. in human factors from the University of Queensland in 2005, specializing in fatigue, workload, and situation awareness in the maritime domain. During her career she was involved in teaching and tutoring in human factors-related topics. Through her academic research work and experience, Michelle has acquired a comprehensive publications list, including refereed journal articles, as well as national and international conference papers. Michelle has also been involved in a number of European Union (EU) maritime safety projects. She is periodically involved as a maritime human factors expert in the evaluation of maritime research projects for the EU Director General of Transport. Michelle, a chartered engineer, has spent most of her career working within the maritime industry in Malta and in Australia starting off as a project engineer, engineering consultant, marine surveyor, and maritime human factors researcher.

Tim Horberry. Tim is associate professor of human factors at the University of Queensland, Australia. Before that, he was head of human factors within the transportation division at the UK Transport Research Laboratory. Dr. Horberry has successfully supervised several Ph.D. students working in the field of transport human factors. He has published his work widely and is a registered member of the UK Ergonomics Society. He coedited another book on transport safety, which was published by CRC Press in 2004.

Thomas Koester. Thomas Koester, psychologist, MA, is employed at FORCE Technology in Kongens Lyngby near Copenhagen. Thomas has during the last seven years worked with applied psychology and human factors in safety-critical domains including maritime transport, power plants, off-shore industry, railroads, and hospitals. Thomas has participated in EU projects and thematic networks about maritime safety and human factors, and he is working with development and teaching of human factors and crew resource management courses for maritime personnel, off-shore personnel, power plant personnel, personnel from the health care sector, and accident investigators. He is cofounder of the Maritime Human Factors Research Group (www.maritimehumanfactors.org), member of Danish Human Factors Centre (www.dhfc.dk), and associated member of Centre for Human–Machine Interaction 2000–2003.

chapter one

Introduction to maritime human factors

1.1 History and development of maritime human factors

1.1.1 Early days: hazards of shipping

To appreciate the importance of the human element within maritime operations, we need to understand how this domain historically has gone about its business. Historical maritime snippets may enlighten us on this issue.

Some of the qualities most valued in mariners prior to mechanically propelled ships included physical strength, endurance, an ability to withstand a high level of discomfort, and to some extent an indifference to pain and even death. This is summed up in Gomes De Brito's translated description of a mariner's life in the fifteenth century.

> Being about to write down the disastrous voyage of this great ship, it occurred to me how rash men are in their undertakings, chief among which, or one of the greatest, was confiding their lives to four planks lashed together, and to the discretion of the furious winds, with which they live in such wise that we can rightly say "quia ventus est vita mea" (my life is like a wind), and thus traverse the vast expanse of the watery element, encompassing the whole earth. (Gomes De Brito, Boxer, and Blackmore 2001)

Shipping, although profitable, was considered a dangerous business in those days and men who traversed the sea were believed to be either reckless or foolish. The ship *Sao Paolo,* referred to as "the great ship" in the above text, foundered off the coast of Sumatra in 1562. This was actually one of several tragic shipwrecks that occurred during the sixteenth and seventeenth centuries on what was then known as the *carreiri da India,* the sea route between Portugal and the Indian subcontinent. This trade route was known to be very profitable, but not without its hazards. It was well recognized as notoriously dangerous. During the period from 1550 to 1650 sources point to losses from shipwrecks reaching "alarming proportions." Most of these shipwrecks occurred on the homeward journey, suggesting that most were overladen with cargo. Information from several sources revealed that the primary causes for the loss of so many *carracks** in the Indian Ocean:

> were mainly due to willful overloading by the officers, passengers and crew, and to the superficial and inadequate careening carried out during the ship's stay at Goa. Contributory causes were inefficient stowage of the cargo; leaving Goa too late in the season; the crankiness of the top heavy four deck carracks; ships in a fleet parting company so as to reach Lisbon first and get a better market for their "private trade"; the mulish obstinacy of some of the pilots; and the inexperience of some gentlemen-commanders. (Gomes De Brito, Boxer, and Blackmore 2001)

Human error, although not mentioned explicitly, had already been identified as one of the primary factors contributing to these casualties. To some extent, there was some kind of control exercised on these "dangerous practices," as they were called in those days. During this period there were so-called standing orders in place that contained stringent rules against "overloading, improper stowage of cargo, abuse of berth and deck space, the enlistment of unqualified mariners, or their substitution by inexperienced men" (Gomes De Brito, Boxer, and Blackmore 2001). These orders were introduced mainly as a curb to the large losses of galleons and their expensive, lavish cargo, rather than as a risk-reduction strategy for preventing any further loss of lives. In addition, a punishable offense was instituted for pilots found guilty of failing to communicate effectively with their colleagues on board. Printed regulations were also distributed to all ships on this route. However, ship losses continued. It was only after 1650 that records point to a sudden drop in shipwrecks. The main reason for this was attributed to the hanging of some ships' officers who were charged with misconduct over the loss of two galleons in the late 1650s. This may perhaps explain why a punitive attitude is still so deeply rooted in the maritime domain, although the domain does not go as far as hanging ships' crew anymore. The perception in this domain, even today, seems to be that punishment works (Chapter 7 provides further discussion on this topic). These hangings actually did act as a deterrent for a short while, dropping the shipwreck toll in line with the English and Dutch ships, which set an average "good" standard for that time. Other nations, such as France, introduced a more regulatory approach. Its measures included ship inspections to ensure that vessels complied with

---

* Carracks were large, three- or four-masted ships, characterized by deep draught, relatively broad beam, and very high fore and aft castles. They carried large cargoes, were in most cases fitted for warfare, and mainly used by the Portuguese in trading with the East Indies. They possessed characteristics similar to galleons.

loading regulations of the time. However, such deterrents were short-lived, with hazard prevention being a more or less rudimentary matter.

1.1.2 1800s to World War II: birth of international ship safety regulations

Up to the mid-1800s, people avoided traveling by sea as much as possible, as it was well known to be a hazardous venture. Navigational aids were virtually non-existent, with mariners relying on crude implements to guide them. Shipboard fires and collisions with icebergs were feared and cited as contributory causes in a large number of ship losses. During the winter of 1820 alone, maritime casualty statistics point to figures of as many as two thousand ships lost in the North Sea. Winter travel was seldom undertaken in the days of the more vulnerable wooden ships, but this changed dramatically with the advent of the "invincible" iron ship.

The 1850s hailed the arrival of iron and steel and steam engines, which provided the technology for the construction of larger, stronger, faster ships, considered to be more controllable and less susceptible to damage. Such technical advances, however, introduced a new breed of hazards. Early steam engines were not without their problems and did tend to explode sometimes, leaving behind huge death tolls. The American steamboat *Sultana* was one such ship. On 27 April 1865, three of its four boilers exploded while traveling on the Mississippi River in Memphis, Tennessee (Potter 1992). An estimated 1,700 of the *Sultana*'s overcrowded 2,400 passengers were either killed in the explosion or drowned when the *Sultana* sank. An official enquiry revealed that the cause of the tragedy was a leaky and poorly repaired steam boiler, exacerbated by the overcrowding, which made the vessel too top heavy. There was much finger pointing as a result of this tragedy; however, in the wake of the assassination of President Abraham Lincoln and the end of the Civil War in the United States at that time, interest in the *Sultana* disaster fizzled.

Maritime safety standards were at best laissez faire in the mid-nineteenth century. Nevertheless, people's perception of sea travel changed dramatically, and by the late 1800s and early 1900s it became one of the most popular modes of travel. Advances in technology opened a market for passenger ships. Maritime transport was at this stage booming, so it was natural for authorities to start exercising at least some kind of control via regulatory national safety standards available at the time, especially because the general population venturing to the sea had extended beyond the typical mariner. This period also heralded the birth of classification societies, which were private organizations that provided information to insurance companies on the quality of ships and their equipment. Accidents and majors disasters encouraged various countries to cooperate more where introduction of certain maritime safety standards was concerned. This sparked the start of a reactive maritime culture in which new safety rules were introduced following major accidents. In 1879, the first joint rules for an international code of signals were adopted by nineteen countries. In 1880 and 1881, the first set of international rules on the "prevention of collisions at sea" and "health and safety" for "steam navigation" were signed. This led to adoption of more rules relating to wireless telegraphy and lifesaving equipment. It was not long after, that safety standards in specific areas were adopted at a rapid pace, especially where passenger travel was concerned. One of the most discussed and well-known tragedies in history initiated a significant campaign toward improved passenger ship safety standards. On April 14, 1912 the *RMS Titanic* struck an iceberg off Newfoundland (Canada) and sank together with 1,500 of its passengers and crew. This tragedy created a media frenzy when the realization dawned that, had the vessel been fitted with adequate safety equipment, the death toll would have been significantly less. This sparked the first International Conference on Safety of Life at Sea held in London in 1914. The conference addressed safety technical issues that came out of the *Titanic* enquiry, such as the adequacy of lifeboats, hull subdivision, and radio communications equipment on passenger ships. World War I, however, kept the 1914 Safety of Life at Sea (SOLAS) Convention at bay for a while, but not for long. The first SOLAS Convention came into force in 1919.

Regrettably, maritime history is plagued with ship accidents and losses such as the *Titanic*, although fortunately not always as severe. Reaction to high-profile accidents has historically resulted in the introduction of new regulatory measures. This trend continues even today within the international maritime community. Recently, however, there has been a shift in this approach and the international maritime community has finally come to realize that being proactive, rather than following a historically reactive approach, is the key to accident prevention.

1.1.3   World War II to the end of the 1960s: beginnings of maritime human factors

World War II created a springboard for specific scientific human factors work, attributable mainly to human limitations becoming more apparent. This, however, was not as a response to the soaring rate of maritime accidents and lives lost at sea. Instead, the requirement for people to perform more effectively was seen as important during time of war. In this regard, an increase in personnel efficiency of between 15 and 35 percent was frequently quoted as a result of scientific studies in human factors conducted during World War II. This provided the impetus for further research work in the area of maritime human factors—it also happened across other domains such as aviation.

Some of the more prominent work in maritime human factors was initiated by the United States with the establishment of the Committee on Undersea Warfare in 1946. A *Panel on Psychology and Physiology* was appointed with a specific mandate to draw up an outline for a number of surveys in applied research on problems related to human factors in undersea warfare. Wartime dictated that most of this work focused mainly on naval vessels. Donald Lindsley, then chairman of the panel, had a pretty good notion of what he wanted to achieve from these surveys.

> In each case there is the problem of whether the task imposed by equipment and the amount of information to be obtained from it is within the range of the capacities of the human individuals using it, whether they can translate the information, interpret it if necessary, and pass it on to controls centers where it can be used to best advantage. (Donald Lindsey, Preface for Panel on Psychology and Physiology, 1949)

Although the outcome of the reports that came out of these surveys focused on submarine issues, the intention was to allow cross transfer of research and development effort to other maritime platforms. The studies focused on such factors as visual and auditory problems, design and arrangement of operating equipment, habitability issues, and selection and training. This work heralded a breakthrough in maritime human factors for the time.

In the beginning of the 1950s, the U.S. Navy commissioned the National Naval Medical Center to conduct research on the ease with which navy recruits adapted themselves to various watch schedules. The main purpose of this research was to establish whether more effective watch schedules could be devised that would provide a marked increase in human performance at sea. This research attempted to identify whether body temperature could be linked to performance (attention). This was one of the first studies in the area of fatigue.

Meanwhile, in Europe, maritime human factors research work had started to focus more on bridge design, this time for merchant ships. The electronic age was creeping in with more sophisticated navigation and communication systems. The introduction of such advances in technology also created the requirement for a new breed of specialist seafarers. Cognitive and specialized technical skills replaced the physical strength and endurance as qualities required of modern mariners. As the structural reliability of ships improved and their ability to survive in adverse environmental conditions increased, the type of operational failures leading to casualties also changed dramatically. The collision between the two passenger ships *Andrea Doria* and the *Stockholm* in 1956 is one such example. This accident, together with many others at the time, was referred to as a typical *radar-assisted* collision. This fired up some interest in the area of bridge design and cognition, both in Europe and the United States. It was during this time that Walraven (1967), who conducted research in the area of human factors and bridge design in the Netherlands, came to realize that most human factors needs in maritime operations were being subsumed by an increase in automation. He developed a mature concept of what he believed maritime human factors should be all about: "design has to be seen as an integrated problem, and not as a number of independent part problems. It is moreover extremely useful to have discussion between builder, user and designer" (Walraven 1967, p. 607).

The 1960s also saw a lot more work done in the area of human fatigue, focusing on the effect of work–rest scheduling and sleep loss on naval crew performance. Apart from the United States, the Royal Navy (RN) Personnel Research Committee in the United Kingdom initiated research efforts in watchkeeping and performance at sea (Colquhoun, Blake, and Edwards 1969). Their research focused on the diurnal rhythm and sleep loss, confirming the time of day effect on fatigue and human performance. This research work is today viewed as a crucial foundation for the ongoing work in the area of fatigue. The International Maritime Organization* (IMO) has also shown a great deal of interest in the area of shipboard fatigue in the last decade. In this regard it has developed fatigue management guidelines specifically for shipboard personnel. The topic of fatigue and performance is discussed more extensively in Chapter 3.

1.1.4   1970s and beyond

During the 1970s, a number of minor human factors initiatives had started to hatch in Europe and the United States. Ship statistics in the 1970s indicated that more than one merchant ship per day was being lost at sea. This started alarm bells ringing, with the result that in the early 1970s the U.S. Maritime Transportation Research Board commissioned research work in the area of *human error*, specifically looking at "providing recommendations that will lead to the development of countermeasures against acts of commission or omission that lead to merchant marine casualties" (Maritime Transportation Research Board 1976, p. 2). Systematic and quantitative historical human error data were found to be lacking; hence collection of data was mainly conducted through the use of questionnaire surveys, utilizing expert judgment for evaluation. These studies identified a number of contributory human factors as either major or potential causes of casualties, and included such factors as "inattention, inefficient bridge design, poor operational procedures, poor eyesight, excessive fatigue, ambiguous pilot–master relationship, excessive alcohol use, excessive personnel turnover, high level of calculated risk, inadequate lights and markers, misuse of radar, uncertain use of sound signals, and inadequacies of the rules and regulations" (Maritime Transportation Research Board 1976, pp. 7–14). Based on these factors, the panel recommended a number of improvements in these areas. These mainly focused on crew error and refrained from looking any further than this.

Throughout the 1980s maritime human factors seemed to pass through a period of darkness where initiatives in this area were few and sparse. However, major maritime accidents still dominated the scene. Unfortunately, it

---

* See Glossary for more information.

had to be a spate of well-known major disasters, such as the huge loss of life in the capsize of the passenger ferries *Herald of Free Enterprise* in 1987 and the *Estonia* in 1994, as well as major oil spills from the oil tankers *Exxon Valdez* in 1989 and the *Braer* in 1993 and many others, that led to a revival in the field of maritime human factors. Perhaps the 1990s can be seen as having reached a maximum number of maritime accidents, fatalities, and environmental pollution such that the public was not able to tolerate any more.

As history dictates, the maritime community continued focusing on developing safety rules as a result of such tragic disasters. One example is the Oil Pollution Act (OPA 90), which came into force in the United States in 1990 following the *Exxon Valdez* disaster. This required the U.S. Coast Guard (USCG) to strengthen its regulations on oil tankers entering U.S. waters. Nevertheless, the beginnings of the 1990s also saw the start of *human factors* definitions being publicized around the global maritime community. The *human error* viewpoint spread like wildfire. Analyses of casualty reports provided a method of somehow quantifying these "vague" human factor issues in such a way as to send the necessary warning signals of the existence of the problem.

In 1993, the USCG reported that 80 percent of maritime accidents were caused by human error. On these grounds, the Prevention through People (PTP) program was initiated, which looked at developing a long-term safety strategy focusing on human error prevention (U.S. Coast Guard 1995). In 1994, a U.K. Protection and Indemnity (P&I) club* study on major P&I claims between 1987 and 1993 indicated that 63 percent of these incidents were caused by human error. In the same year the IMO reported that more than 75 percent of ship accidents worldwide were due to human error. In this regard, the IMO recommended that the study of human factors (and in particular human error) would be an important focus for improving maritime safety. As a result, although initially largely reactive in its response, the IMO started to focus on introducing new regulations that incorporated a *human element* viewpoint. Examples include the International Safety Management (ISM) code and the revised Standards for Training, Certification and Watchkeeping for Seafarers (STCW) Convention. The ISM code was adopted in an attempt to curb poor management practices in international shipping, which are discussed further in Chapter 7. The revised STCW Convention was adopted in 1995 and entered into force in 1997. This convention incorporated a new set of requirements for minimum training standards and competency for seafarers. Whether these codes have been effective or not in improving safety at sea is still being debated today. What is certain, however, is that the IMO was perceived as tackling the human error concern.

The 1990s also saw an increase in application of human systems engineering (HSE) within the U.S. Navy, which included more than just traditional HSE elements. This incorporated such applications as comfort and crew

---

* See Glossary for definition.

safety and the incorporation of optimal crew numbers to maximize total system performance in operating and maintaining the system. The USCG also commenced developing a similar initiative in the mid-1990s referred to as human systems integration (HSI) as part of the planning, design, and development of its system acquisition process. In principle, the general approach used for HSI in the United States is that it relates to five domains: human factors engineering; crewing; personnel; training; and system safety. These domains are viewed as connected during system acquisition. Today, HSI principles have gone a long way within the maritime sector. The U.S. and U.K. navies have some of the most mature maritime human systems (or factors) integration models in place. Merchant shipping is adopting a similar approach and has opted for a more customized model referred to as the sociotechnical network model. This book is mainly based on the sociotechnical network model, discussed further in later sections.

Today, there have been substantial developments in the area of human factors in the maritime domain. In the last few years, Maritime Human Factors (MHF) research groups have been set up in Europe and the United States to discuss and collaborate on their research findings. A number of MHF initiatives are already providing some valuable information and insight into the area of human factors. One such initiative is the International Maritime Human Element Forum, a Nautical Institute (international professional body for qualified mariners) project sponsored by one of the major classification societies, Lloyds Register of Shipping, with the aim of improving human element awareness in the maritime domain.

We have now moved beyond the second millennium and perhaps it is fair to ask whether human factors skills and knowledge in the maritime domain have been adequately applied in the past and what can be done to ensure adequate progresses for the future. We hope that this book will provide a basis upon which a reasoned assessment can be made.

1.2   Complexity of commercial shipping

Perhaps it is appropriate at this stage to provide a brief overview of shipping in general, to understand the difficulties and issues that arise because of its international character and complexity. This should provide a basis for recognition of the human factors challenges that face this particular industry.

In spite of developments that have taken place in other forms of transport, such as air and road transport, the sea remains one of the most important connecting links between the nations. More than three quarters of world trade volume is moved by sea. Advances in design and construction technology have encouraged development of ship types that can satisfy growing economic demands, and this includes greater capacity, faster speeds, and more turnarounds. In line with these aims, a ship is designed, built, and operated to maximize its total cargo transportation capacity, whether carrying goods or passengers.

1.2.1   Organizational change in shipping

Up to the early post-war (WWII) years, world shipping was dominated by the fleets of the traditional maritime nations: the United Kingdom, the United States, France, Netherlands, and the Scandinavian countries, to cite but a few examples. However, from the 1950s onward a gradual change took place in the fleet distribution. The traditional maritime nations were no longer dominating the world tonnage figures. This was caused to some extent by a diversion of resources from the maritime sector resulting in a reduced amount of investment, but perhaps more significantly by the flight to the open registries, better known as *flags of convenience*. A large number of shipping companies started changing the country of registry of their vessels from the traditional countries to these open registries. Attractiveness of these open registries stemmed from the fact that they provided benefits such as tax allowances. They also introduced a globalization factor into the picture—allowing employment of ships' crew hailing from developing countries (other than that of the flag state). By 1999, about half of all registered merchant ships flew flags of convenience. There has been a lot of criticism over the years of this system, mainly related to safety issues. A negative global image was being created of these open registries as flags with low safety standards that allowed any rust bucket on the verge of sinking to be registered. There is continual dispute on this issue; however, what is certain is that open registries dominate the world tonnage figures and are here to stay.

While open registries are one phenomenon that points to a fundamental shift in the organization of international maritime transport, another one relates to ship management. A growing spurt in the shipping sector during the 1990s influenced more ship owners to hand over responsibility for ship operations to professional ship management organizations, a trend that had started during the 1980s. A very substantial portion of the international commercial fleet is today managed under such arrangements. The vessel situation became such that the owner could be located in one country, the ship management company located in a second country, and same vessel could be registered in a third country. It has thus become difficult to identify the true ownership of, and for that matter the accountability for, many vessels engaged in commercial shipping. The flag flown and the port of registry do not any longer reveal conclusive evidence of ownership. Maritime transport has become a very complex industry indeed.

1.2.2   The regulatory aspect

The international nature of the shipping industry has led to action being taken to improve safety in maritime operations, which is now enforced at the international level. This complexity is further increased by the influence of national and international regulations adopted by local and international bodies, notably the IMO, the International Labour Organization (ILO), as well as by the most influential classification societies. The IMO was established as a permanent international body to promote maritime safety more effectively, and started off by adopting a new version of SOLAS, the most important of all treaties dealing with maritime safety. The IMO is made up of government departments and agencies from all over the world with a particular interest in shipping. These government departments and agencies usually regulate ship operation and safety under the IMO umbrella. Such agencies are also empowered to regulate environmental aspects of shipping under the Maritime Pollution (MARPOL) Convention. Today, the most important international conventions dealing with maritime safety, such as SOLAS and MARPOL, have been widely accepted and applied to more than 95 percent of the world's merchant shipping fleet. This means that it would be almost impossible to operate a ship that does not meet IMO agreed requirements or standards.

In theory, the universal application of IMO instruments would ensure that casualty rates would be virtually the same for all flags. However, this is obviously not the case. From available statistics, ships operating under the flag administration with the worst casualty record are more likely to have an accident than those with the best record. This disturbing fact may be attributed to cultural differences in the national implementation and enforcement of IMO requirements.

The introduction of *Port State Control* by the IMO has to some extent brought some level of control over substandard ships. This control empowered coastal states to inspect and detain any merchant ship visiting their ports which they believed to be substandard.* Hence, in addition to international regulations, ships are subject to the laws of various countries that they visit in the course of their business. In this case, the ships are said to be under the jurisdiction of the port or the coastal state.

1.2.3   The classification aspect

Apart from the regulatory authorities such as the IMO, some aspects of ship design, construction, and maintenance standards are also covered by classification society standards, which have been accepted as semiofficial bodies in major maritime nations. Classification societies develop technical rules, regulations, standards, and guidelines dealing with associated ship surveys and inspections covering the design, construction, and through-life compliance of a ship. Contrary to IMO conventions, classification is purely voluntary for ship owners; the only penalty that can be imposed for noncompliance with classification rules is suspension or cancellation of the classification notation. However, there is a Catch 22 in all this. When a ship is submitted for insurance and registration purposes, underwriters and ship registers require a guarantee

---

* Substandard refers to not meeting IMO convention requirements relating to maritime safety and pollution prevention. This also incorporates ILO standards relating to crew accommodation and conditions on board.

that the vessel is structurally sound for the intended service, so that almost all trading vessels usually go through the classification process. Classification also provides a crucial contribution to the international shipping community in terms of technical support and compliance verification, backed by relevant research and development. In reality, most government administrations (flag states) responsible for implementing the IMO conventions often delegate these responsibilities to classification societies. Classification societies have a very good network of regional offices in all major, and most minor, shipping centers around the world and they are the natural choice, given their expertise, knowledge, and global presence, to provide this service.

1.3   Human factors

As we have seen in earlier parts of this chapter, consideration of human factors is becoming increasingly important in the maritime domain. Before we delve further into the subject of human factors, we first must start by presenting a comprehensible definition to provide a better understanding of its scope.

There are a number of human factors definitions around in various textbooks and publications ultimately leading to the same theme. For example, the International Ergonomics Association provides the following definition:

> Ergonomics (or human factors) is the scientific discipline concerned with the understanding of the interactions among humans and other elements of a system, and the profession that applies theory, principles, data and methods to design in order to optimise human well being and overall system performance. (International Ergonomics Association)

Over the years there have also been some misunderstandings on the use and definitions of terminologies such as *human factors* and *ergonomics*, which essentially have similar meanings. The term *human factors* is more commonly applied in the United States, whereas *ergonomics*, which comes from the Greek words *ergon* (work) and *nomos* (natural law), is preferred in Europe.

To avoid any confusion or ambiguity in this area the IMO has recently opted for the use of the words *human element* as an alternative. IMO Resolution A.947 (23) published in February 2004 lays down the "Human Element Vision, Principles and Goals for the Organization." The IMO perhaps perceives this to be a helpful alternative without causing too much anguish to the Americans and Europeans.

Whatever the name, a vital element of all this is the notion of *fit* between the person(s) and their surrounding environment. That is, fitting the task, equipment, or environment to the capabilities and limitations of person(s), rather than trying to adapt or fit the person(s) to the tasks and running the risk of forcing them to operate unsuitable or poorly designed equipment or work systems. Essentially, Vincente (2004) indicates: "If the human factor is taken into account, a tight fit between person and design can be achieved and the technology is more likely to fulfill its intended purpose" (Vincente 2004, p. 54). Hence, underlying the subject is the idea that using human factors data, principles, and methods will lead to better designed jobs, tasks, products, or work systems. This in turn will have benefits, both for individuals (through improved well-being) and employers (through improving work performance of individuals and groups in an organization).

1.3.1   Human factors and the maritime domain

To set the scene for this section we first need to provide a brief description of the work on board ships. Despite the various ship types out there, the maritime work domain can in broad terms be defined as any kind of work performed on board any kind of vessel. According to the European BERTRANC project (BERTRANC 2000) it is possible to define five maritime work tasks:

1. Navigation: Route planning, track keeping, and collision avoidance
2. Propulsion: The responsibility for the integrity of the ship's propulsion system and associated auxiliaries
3. Cargo handling: Loading, keeping the cargo (including passengers) in good condition, and unloading
4. Platform maintenance: Keeping the ship, its equipment (e.g., the auxiliary equipment), and the crew (the hotel function) in operational condition
5. Ship management: Allocation of tasks and responsibilities, control and supervision, and communication

In many ways, the ship also presents an unusual and sometimes very harsh work environment. Crewmembers are required to perform most of their tasks in a moving environment. In addition, the work environment is also characterized by lack of contact with family, by different cultures living together, and for the most part of the job by a high element of boredom. It is no surprise then that this environment itself enhances the risk of errors.

In spite of this, the U.K. P&I Club indicates that human error is declining marginally along the lines of ship losses,* which over the last decade have been steadily decreasing. Figure 1.1 charts ship losses from 1996 to 2004 for the entire global maritime industry and provides an indication of this level of improvement. In spite of this, however, the human factor continues to play a major role in accident and incident causation, accounting for 58 percent of major P&I claims. Hence, similar to other transport domains, it seems that human performance problems constitute a significant threat to system safety. As indicated, there are a number of factors within the maritime work

---

* A "loss" refers to ships damaged beyond economic repair.

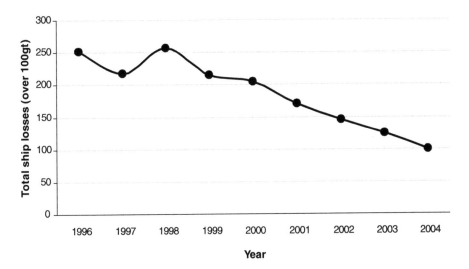

Figure 1.1 Total ship losses by number (ships over 100 gt). Reproduced with permission from Lloyd's Register Fairplay.

domain that could positively or negatively influence human performance at sea. Some of the most influential include:

- Crewing numbers
- New technology
- Crew demographics
- Social factors

It should be noted that this is not an exhaustive list, but it does form a good foundation, as it serves as a basis for the rest of this book. Each of these factors is discussed briefly below using some maritime examples.

1.3.1.1 Crewing numbers

On 29 June 2003, the general cargo vessel *Jambo* ran aground and subsequently sank off the west coast of Scotland. The single-hold vessel was carrying 3,300 tons of zinc concentrate, prompting fears of a major environmental disaster. This accident was the latest of a series of similar accidents in which common features included one man bridge operation at night leading to fatigue, prompting some level of awareness on the crewing issue in the maritime community.

In the last decade there has been a worldwide trend to reduce the amount of human labor; the shipping sector has not escaped this trend. Although twenty or so years ago ships were staffed with crew complements of between forty to fifty people, it is not uncommon today to have larger tankers and cargo ships with an average crew size of twenty people or fewer. Figure 1.2 shows the average full crew numbers by size and type of ship for a sample

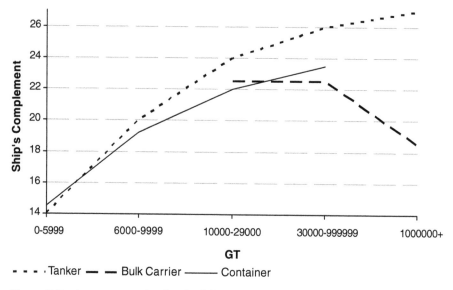

Figure 1.2 Average crewing levels (2002 to 2004) on U.K. P&I Club ships by size/ type of ship. Reproduced with permission from the United Kingdom Mutual Steam Ship Assurance Association (Bermuda) Limited (the U.K. P&I Club).

of 197 tankers, 433 bulk carriers, and 193 container ships. Crewing numbers have more than halved from a decade ago.

It is today a mandatory requirement, through the reference in SOLAS, for merchant vessels to carry a minimum safe manning certificate. The IMO Resolution A.890 (21) (Annex B) provides some guidance regarding this SOLAS requirement, which takes into account size, operational profile, and technical equipment of the vessel. Although these guidelines are relatively comprehensive, the final decision regarding minimum crew size is usually based on a subjective assessment by the relevant administration (flag state). This may sometimes be subject to some pressure from ship owners and operators, whose main goal is to reduce operational costs, compelling certain administrations to be somewhat lenient in their final decision, rather than losing revenue through loss of ship registrations.

A review of existing certificates and a comparison with actual operational requirements on board indicate that crew numbers are often insufficient to properly address specific onboard tasks (such as loading/unloading, maintenance, emergency response, or mooring/unmooring) without violating minimum rest period requirements or introducing potential human performance decrements. Studies conducted by the U.K. Maritime Accident Investigation Bureau (MAIB) on collisions, groundings, and contacts between 1994 and 2003 highlighted a link between crew numbers and ship accidents (Marine Accident Investigation Branch 2001a). This study acknowledges that crew numbers for watchkeeping personnel on board are often inadequate, which in most cases leads to fatigue (e.g., leading to a failure to maintain a good lookout).

The cost factor has also created situations where ships' turnaround time has been reduced drastically when compared to, for example, thirty years ago. Back then, crew used time ashore for respite and recovery; in some cases there would have been enough time for their families to visit while the ship was unloading at berth. Today, containerization of vessels has meant that container ships dock at special terminals far away from towns or cities and spend very little time berthed. In this case crewmembers need to stay on board as loading and unloading times do not provide time for the crew to wander ashore anymore. This shorter turnaround time, combined with reduced crew size, constrains crewmembers to stay on board the vessel and continue working, restricting and contravening rest periods. This has an influence on crew fatigue and stress factors, which today have been recognized as causal factors in a number of maritime accidents. Chapter 2 and Chapter 3 will provide further insight to these issues from a human factors perspective.

1.3.1.2 New technology

Traditionally the international maritime community has approached maritime safety from a predominantly technical perspective. It was common practice to apply engineering and technological solutions such as radar, ARPA (Automated Radar Plotting Aid), and GPS (Global Positioning System) to promote safety and minimize the risks of accidents. The human element aspect was treated in a peripheral manner, with little or no consideration given to human and organizational errors. Despite the progress made in advancing technology, systems have not yet been developed that are immune to errors committed by those who operate them. To illustrate the case, the collision between the two passenger ships *Andrea Doria* and the *Stockholm* in 1956, referred to previously, provides a good example of the role of *technology* in error causation. In this tragic event, fifty-one people lost their lives, and the passenger liner *Andrea Doria* sank as a result. Although this event happened some time ago, it was at a time where significant developments were being made in radar technology. This "new" technology had started to form an integral part of merchant ships' navigational systems. The *Andrea Doria* was equipped with two of the latest radar scopes, and in addition there were three experienced officers on the bridge at the time of the collision. A question has been asked many times: "How it was possible that two great ocean liners, manned by experienced crews and having the latest 1950s radar technology, could collide in open waters?" The third officer was on watch on the *Stockholm* at the time of the collision. Both vessels were traveling at high speed (twenty-one knots for the *Andrea Doria* and eighteen knots for the *Stockholm*) in calm but foggy conditions. The navigating officers of both the *Andre Doria* and the *Stockholm* were relying entirely on radar outputs to verify their vessels' position in relation to their surroundings. Although the third officer of the *Stockholm* did detect the *Andrea Doria* on his radar scope he mistakenly used the wrong radar range, resulting in a misinterpretation of the closest point of approach (CPA). This finally led to the inevitable, with the *Stockholm* literarily ramming the *Andrea Doria*'s side. This event led to significant changes to the IMO collision regulations with an emphasis on ships' speed in low-visibility conditions. However, the main problem of *how* and *why* did the third officer of the *Stockholm* mistakenly use the wrong scale on the radar was never really questioned. So, although most accidents involving collisions point toward a breach in the IMO collision regulations, a number of studies reveal shortfalls in the human element. This emphasizes the need to design and develop new technology that meets overall system requirements, but also accounts for human limitations within that system. The interaction between technology and the individual is further discussed in Chapter 6.

1.3.1.3   *Crew demographics and social factors*

It is not uncommon for a ship to have crew hailing from different countries, speaking different languages, and coming from diverse cultural and social backgrounds. There are a number of reasons for this shift in crew demographics. First, as discussed earlier the introduction of open registries set the scene for the employment of seafarers from different nationalities. Second, a seafaring career today is not looked on as favorably as it was thirty or so years ago. This could be the result of deteriorating crew conditions, short-term career prospects, and lack of opportunities when compared to shore-based jobs, with the consequence that people, especially those coming from the more traditional seafaring nations, have been discouraged to seek seagoing careers. Another reason is once again a consequence of economics. To reduce costs, ship owners and ship operators are hiring crew from countries offering much lower wages and willing to accept poorer working conditions. This situation has created many challenges to shipboard crew. For starters, although communication issues have always had a niggling presence in ships' officer–pilot interaction component, today it is not uncommon to have language and communication problems present even between crew of the same ship. English is today widely accepted as the language at sea, and this has been accounted for within the STCW Convention. However, language problems today still play a contributory part in human and organizational error. These are actually some of the specific risk areas that the U.K. P&I Club has identified as causes of human error. Such communication problems also extend to interfacing issues between shipboard and shoreside personnel, both from within the company and also from dockside workers such as stevedores, etc. As is the trend globally, the use of multinational crew has also weakened, to some extent, company loyalty, perhaps adding another dimension, apart from the language barrier, to human factors issues on board, such as the seafarer attitudes, safety culture, and behavior toward their job. Most of the human factors aspects described in this section are covered in more detail in Chapter 4 and Chapter 7.

1.4   Accidents and human error

1.4.1   The accident pyramid

A large number of maritime accidents and incidents involve some form of human error as we will see in later chapters. Studies show that for each serious accident in the maritime domain, or in any other domain, there are a larger number of incidents, an even larger number of near-misses, and many more safety-critical events and unsafe acts. Figure 1.3 depicts this classis *iceberg* model, showing accidents as the tip, near-misses as the base, and incidents as the center. A number of studies have confirmed this pyramidal relationship between the categories, with ratios varying according to the type of industry. If incidents and near-miss data are well understood, they can provide important clues to ways a system is able to recover and revert to a safe state. As in Figure 1.3, the accident pyramid goes beyond the near-misses base. Frequent but almost invisible, potentially dangerous unsafe acts and everyday work routines, with a safety-critical potential, occur in much larger numbers than near misses and these lie closer to the foundation of the pyramid. This means that by focusing only on accidents, incidents, and near misses we are concentrating only on the tip of the iceberg, thereby missing out on a large amount of everyday work routines, actions, and behavioral data. Even so, there is an increasing realization that a systematic analysis of minor incidents and near-miss data can yield a great amount of reliable information that can be used to improve safety. Domains such as aviation and medicine have implemented such systems, which have been in place for years and are already retrieving valuable information. The maritime domain has just started implementing such reporting systems, including the Maritime Accident Investigation Branch (MAIB) in the United Kingdom and the U.S. Coast Guard. In spite of these

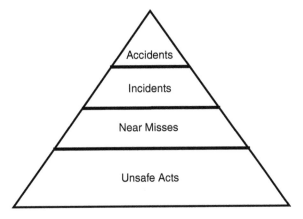

Figure 1.3   The classic iceberg model depicting accidents as the tip and near misses, which occur in much greater numbers, as the base.

initiatives, incident and near-miss reports in the maritime domain remain at present quantitatively and qualitatively insufficient.

1.4.2   *The human error concept*

As in the aviation and other transportation domains, human error is at the root of most preventable casualties in the maritime field. Sanders and McCormick (1993) define human error as "an inappropriate or undesirable human decision or behavior that reduces—or has potential for reducing system effectiveness, safety or performance" (p. 606). It is well known that humans regularly make mistakes, and as a consequence human error has stimulated the interest of many cognitive psychologists and system engineers in the last decade. The maritime domain's assertion that the majority of mishaps are due to human error (in some form) is consistent with all other safety-critical industries. To some extent it has made human error quantifiable. We know we have a problem, so how do we tackle it? The issue, however, is that these high human error rates fail to account for the complex interactions that exist between humans and various other contributory factors that lead to system breakdowns; neither do they directly predict future errors. These human errors do not simply occur in isolation, they are intermixed with other problems. To some extent these percentages hide the wide diversity of human errors that occur in the field with the risk that *interventions* or *countermeasures* may fail because they are targeting the wrong type of errors. Details of why certain tasks, equipment, and working environments and their interactions are more susceptible to errors than others are hidden under this huge looming umbrella of human error terminology. There is no learning process involved by referring to human error as a cause. Often the concept of human error leads to the conclusion that the intervention should be directed towards the human operator (e.g., more training, better education, improved selection of personnel, or even punishment or disciplinary actions). But often the problem is not related to the specific individual. Hence, to understand what human error is all about we need to understand the contribution that human factors make to system success and safety. Dekker (2002) provides what he calls a *new view* of human error, which involves three important factors:

- Human error is not a cause of failure. It is the effect, or symptom, of deeper trouble.
- Human error is not random. It is systematically connected to features of people's tools, tasks, and operating environment.
- Human error is not the conclusion of an investigation. It is the starting point. (p. 61)

So where does this leave us? The sociotechnical model, which is described in this chapter, can be applied to solve this dilemma. Let's first have a look at what we mean by this sociotechnical system model.

1.5 The sociotechnical system model

1.5.1 Why a sociotechnical system model?

Historically, humans have developed a divisional approach to solve problems, rather than a more holistic systematic approach. This is reasonable enough as dividing a problem into smaller parts can make it simpler and hence easier to solve. Does it really? Vicente (2004) argues that this "reductionist strategic approach" that has been adopted for centuries by humans has "led directly to our troubles with technology." Vincente mainly attributes this to the fact that scientific knowledge has been divided into two broad groups: the first is the technological sciences, and the second the human sciences. This has created a situation in which most people would be biased toward their own discipline and are usually induced to make the assumption that anything beyond their realm of understanding can be safely ignored. Hence, a situation has arisen where engineers and designers tend to focus only on the technical aspects of design adopting, as Vicente argues, a "mechanistic" view, while the human sciences group tend to focus mainly on people, adopting what he describes as a more "humanistic" view. Vicente provides a threefold, rather pessimistic, set of observations on the pattern of technological problems:

- Technical stuff is frequently too complex for people to manage, creating confusion at best and potentially devastating consequences at worst;
- "Softer" aspects of technological systems (work schedules, team coordination, and so on) can also make people's lives more difficult than they need to be, contributing to chaos; and
- Problems with technology are getting worse, not better. (p. 33)

What Vicente and other human factors experts have been trying to spell out for years is that most designs and technological solutions do not adequately address human capabilities and limitations, that is, the concept of a good fit has not been accounted for. "Design needs to include not just knowledge of the physical world, but knowledge of human being as well" (Vicente 2004, p. 45). More attention needs to focus on the people/technology *relationship* as this influences both human and societal needs. "Doing so should lead to a seamless integration of people and technology, eliminating the bad fits that are causing so much trouble" (Vicente 2004, p. 45). This is what the sociotechnical system model aims to achieve.

1.5.2 Maritime organizations and the sociotechnical system

During the 1960s a number of social scientists at the Tavistock Institute in London formed the idea that organizations could be described as *sociotechnical systems*. Furnham (1997) describes sociotechnical systems as "a set of interrelated elements that functions as a unit for a specific purpose" (p. 74). It is obvious that organizations in the maritime domain are consistent with the sociotechnical systems perspective. As described in previous sections a maritime organization could be the ship owner or shipping company and a part of the organization could be a specific ship. It should also be obvious that ships can be analyzed as a combination of technology (the vessel, engine, equipment, instruments, etc.) and a social system (the crew, their culture, norms, habits, custom, practices, etc.). If we use the idea about sociotechnical systems as an approach for the analysis of maritime accidents and safety we could talk about system error rather than organizational or human error. If we are able to define the "set of interrelated elements" in the sociotechnical system, and thereby build a model of the system, we would have a useful tool for the analysis of maritime accidents, incidents, or safety-related issues, a tool that would be more precise than the general and all-encompassing human error term.

1.5.3 Development of the sociotechnical system model

The sociotechnical system model advocates a more holistic systematic approach rather than a piecemeal, fragmented approach for dealing with relationships among various elements that form a system. But let us go back a few steps before we delve into the sociotechnical system model and provide some insight on the origins of this model.

The well-known SHEL model, originally developed by Edwards (1972) and Hawkins (1987), was actually the starting point that led to the development of the sociotechnical model. The SHEL model describes a system made up of interactions between human (so-called liveware), technology (so-called hardware), procedures (so-called software), and work environment (called the environment). It provides four sets of interactions with the liveware, which represents the central human component, and these include: (1) liveware–liveware, (2) liveware–software, (3) liveware–hardware, and (4) liveware–environment.

The basis of the SHEL model has been used as a framework in the development of a number of taxonomies, namely, the ECCAIRS Explanatory Factors taxonomy used by the International Civil Aviation Organization (ICAO) as an industry standard tool in the analysis of aviation accidents worldwide. This is actually one of the most detailed, comprehensive, and advanced human factors taxonomy in use today. The SHEL model is also in use within the maritime domain where it has been incorporated into IMO Resolution A.884, which provides guidance for maritime accident investigations. Accordingly, although the SHEL model has had a significant impact on human factors principles and processes and has some clear advantages (e.g., its wide use and acceptance and its simple and intuitive feel), it also has some serious shortcomings. The difficulties are mainly associated with the meaning of concepts used in the model, such as hardware, software, and liveware, which can be hard to interpret and communicate. This is more so of a problem today where most common computer users do not make clear distinctions between software and hardware to the same degree as when the model was initially developed in the 1970s and 1980s. This is partly due to the improved user interface of computers. This could be a barrier to the application of the model because, if it is difficult to understand the various metaphors that form the model, it will be difficult to use the model in any given context. Hence, improvements to the SHEL model were undertaken to enhance interpretation and also to create a customized model usable within the maritime domain. This eventually led to the development of what we refer to now as the sociotechnical system model (Koester 2007).

Figure 1.4 shows the current generation of the sociotechnical system model. The dimensions that form part of the model were transformed into a system to create a link between the various concepts. These connections represent "a set of interrelated elements that functions as a unit for a specific purpose" (Furnham 1997), as described previously. This finally leads us to what we refer to now as the sociotechnical system model.

Table 1.1 was created to illustrate how the elements (or nodes) of the sociotechnical model are related to the original categories of the SHEL model. It also provides definitions of the various concepts that form part of the model, some extracted from the SHEL model and some from the ECCAIRS framework.

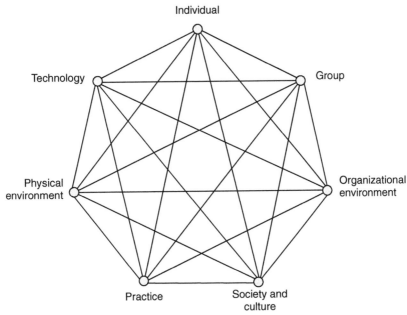

Figure 1.4 The sociotechnical sysem model. The model is also called "The Septigon Model." Septigon refers to Society and Culture, Physical Environment, Practice, Technology, Individual, Group and Organizational Environment Network. Septigon is also the name of a shape with seven sides — the outline of the model. (Koester 2007).

Table 1.1 Connection between SHEL Definitions and Categories Used in the Sociotechnical System Model, Including Definitions of Elements of the Sociotechnical System Categories

SHEL Categories and Definitions[a]	SHEL Categories Breakdown	Sociotechnical System Categories	Definitions from ECCAIRS Explanatory Factors Classification System
Software represents any component such as the policies, norms, rules, procedures, practices, and any other formal or informal rules that define the way the different components of the system interact among themselves and with the external environment	Practice Informal rules Policies Norm Formal rules Procedures	Practice Organizational environment	Custom and practice "... not related to written procedures/ instructions"[b] Company and management[c] procedures[d]
Hardware represents any physical and nonhuman component of the system, such as equipment, vehicles, tools, manuals, signs	Equipment Vehicles Tools Manuals Signs	Technology	Human and hardware interface Inadequate information/data sources Human software/ firmware interface Automation/ automatic systems Automatic defenses/warnings Operational material
Liveware represents human components in their relational and communicational aspects	Human components	Individual	Personal physical or sensory limitations Human physiology Psychological limitations Personal workload management Experience, knowledge, and recency

Table 1.1 Connection between SHEL Definitions and Categories Used in the Sociotechnical System Model, Including Definitions of Elements of the Sociotechnical System Categories (Continued)

SHEL Categories and Definitions[a]	SHEL Categories Breakdown	Sociotechnical System Categories	Definitions from ECCAIRS Explanatory Factors Classification System
	Relational and communicational aspects	Group	Communication Interactions/team skills crew/team resource management training Supervision Regulatory activities[e] Other
Environment represents the sociopolitical and economic environment in which the different components of a process interact	Socio-political and economic environment	Society and culture	Regulatory issues
NA[f]	NA	Physical environment	Physical environment[g]

a According to Rizzo and Save (1999).
b This is part of the explanation of the "custom and practice" category.
c This includes, according to ECCAIRS, company/commercial pressures, specific company problems, management/supervision problems, and personnel policies.
d Procedures are mentioned as part of the system support category in ECCAIRS.
e Regulatory activities according to ECCAIRS include interaction between individuals related to, for example, certification, inspections, monitoring, surveillance, audits, and checks.
f NA, not applicable.
g According to ECCAIRS, this includes weather/visibility conditions, obstructions to vision, physical workspace environment (air quality, temperature, lighting conditions, noise, smoke/fumes, vibration, and anthropometric space).

1.5.4   The Sociotechnical System Model

To complete this first chapter, and to set the scene for subsequent chapters, we expand on the sociotechnical system concept. We argue that the sociotechnical system model is a systematic approach for viewing human factors; it indicates how various factors interact to influence system performance. By managing these factors we can strive to ensure that the system as a whole operates within a safe boundary.

As in Figure 1.4 the sociotechnical model comprises seven main domains:

- Individual
- Practice
- Technology
- Group
- Physical environment
- Organizational environment
- Society and culture

Definitions for these elements originate from Rizzo and Save (1999) and the ECCAIRS Human Factors classification system, as described in Table 1.1. The *individual* refers to the human component, and incorporates such aspects as individual physical or sensory limitations, human physiology, psychological limitations, individual workload management and experience, skill, and knowledge. Some aspects of these individual factors are covered in Chapter 2.

Group refers to the relational and communication aspects, such as communication, interactions, team skills, crew/team resource management training, supervision, and regulatory activities (according to the ECCAIRS framework, regulatory activities cover the interaction between individuals related to aspects such as certification, inspections, monitoring, surveillance, audits, and checks). The group factor, which is also the individual–individual interaction factor, deals with such issues as leadership, communication, and teamwork and is covered in Chapter 4. Some aspects of teamwork will also be dealt with under the organizational–individual interaction factors in Chapter 7.

Technology, according to Rizzo and Save (1999), refers to equipment, vehicles, tools, manuals, and signs. The ECCAIRS framework goes further by also defining technology as the human–hardware interface, information–data sources, human software–firmware interface, automation/automatic systems, automatic defenses/warnings, and operational material. The interaction between technology and the individual, which deals with such factors as equipment, tools, usability, and human machine interaction issues, is examined in more detail in Chapter 6.

Practice refers to such aspects as informal rules and customs. It should, however, be noted that these are not related to written procedures or instructions. Procedures and rules are products of the organization; hence, within the sociotechnical model, these are positioned under the distinct category organizational environment. The interaction between the individual and practice, which deals with the way crew acquire knowledge of the system through practice, is covered in Chapter 7.

The *physical environment*, which refers to the surrounding working environment, includes such aspects as weather/visibility conditions, obstructions to vision, and physical workspace environment (such as air quality, temperature, lighting conditions, noise, smoke/fumes, vibration, ship motion, and anthropometric space). The physical environment–individual interaction factors such as noise vibration, temperature, and ship motion are dealt with in Chapter 5, while other aspects of the physical environment/individual factors such as workspace, work demands, and anthropometry are covered in Chapter 3.

The *organizational environment* refers to company and management and includes such factors as procedures, policies, norms, and formal rules. *Society and culture* refers to the sociopolitical and economic environment in which the organization operates. Both the organizational environment and society and culture factors are covered under Chapter 7.

The next section provides a description of some of the features of the sociotechnical system model by looking at ways it can be applied within the maritime domain, using a passenger ferry situation as an example.

1.5.5 Application of the sociotechnical system model

The photograph in Figure 1.5 shows the captain conducting a tight maneuver in harbor using a joystick. This is a typical example of a relation between the individual (the captain) and technology (joystick). The way this is done is by

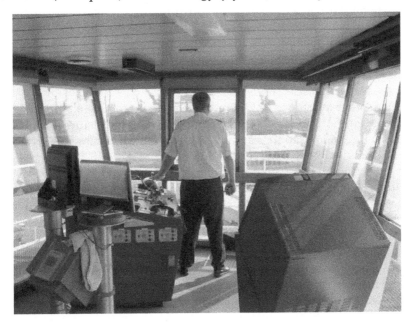

Figure 1.5 The captain maneuvering the vessel from the bridge.

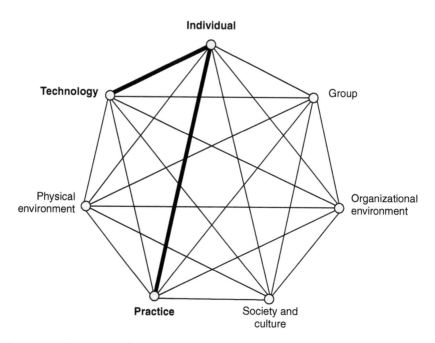

Figure 1.6 Overview of interrelations between specific dimensions as they relate to Figure 1.5.

practice. The group (the crew) is still on the ship (or present in the situation somewhere). All elements in the model are present on at least a residual level, but only some of them are in special focus. In this case it is the individual, technology, and practice. The interactions that are evident in this case are the individual–technology and the individual–practice. Figure 1.6 provides an overview of these interrelations with thick lines used as notations to illustrate the particular case.

The photograph shown in Figure 1.7 demonstrates the same situation, but with one significant difference. The group is now in the picture (the officer is on the bridge talking to the captain). All other elements are still present on at least a residual level; however, as illustrated in Figure 1.7 the following are in focus: individual (the captain), group (the captain and officer), technology (joystick), and practice. The captain still has his hands on the joystick; the officer is not touching anything at this stage. There is therefore no special emphasis on the relation between group and practice. The officer is standing by ready, but he is not performing at the moment. Figure 1.8 provides a representation of this.

This same example can be viewed from a second perspective by changing the focus from the captain to the officer resulting in: individual (officer), group (officer and captain), technology, and practice. Note that in this particular case there would be an interaction between group and technology, which is different from Figure 1.8 where the interaction is between individual and

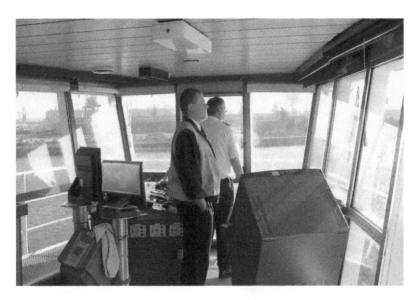

Figure 1.7 The captain and the officer on the bridge.

technology. The interactions formed between the elements are also different. As indicated the interaction between individual and group would probably be communication, and the interaction between individual and technology could be characterized as manual control.

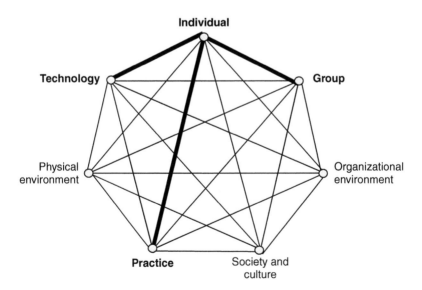

Figure 1.8 Overview of interrelations between specific dimensions as they relate to Figure 1.7.

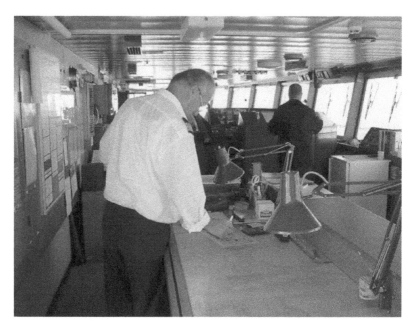

Figure 1.9   The officer fills in a checklist on the bridge during a boat drill.

The next example illustrates the interaction factors involved in conducting a boat drill. In Figure 1.9 the officer is filling out the boat drill checklist on the bridge while crewmembers are conducting the boat drill on the boat deck. The focus in this case is on individual, practice, and organization. We can see from the definition of the various elements in the sociotechnical system model that checklists are part of the organizational environment. Figure 1.10 illustrates the boat drill as seen from the boat deck. Crewmembers swing the boat out ready for launching. Relevant elements from the sociotechnical system model are individual (crewmember), group (crew), technology (the boat and equipment), organizational environment (procedures for the job), and practice (the way the job is actually done, which can differ from how it is described in the procedure). The two photographs in Figure 1.9 and Figure 1.10 are both part of the same event—the boat drill. The two situations illustrated are happening simultaneously but at different locations on the ship: the first one on the bridge, the second on the boat deck. In this case it would make sense to integrate them within the same system seen from the perspective of the officer.

Figure 1.11 shows the boat drill from two perspectives: (1) the bridge, and (2) the boat deck. The constellation of the elements in the system can be explained as follows:

- The officer [individual] is communicating with the crew [group] using the radio [technology].

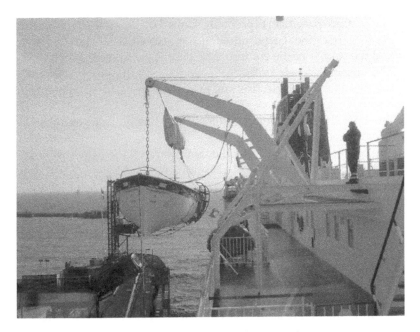

Figure 1.10 A boat drill on the deck. Crewmembers test the equipment.

- The crew [group] is handling the boat [technology].
- Both the crew [group] and the officer [individual] are working in conformity with the checklist [organizational environment] and how the work is usually done [practice].

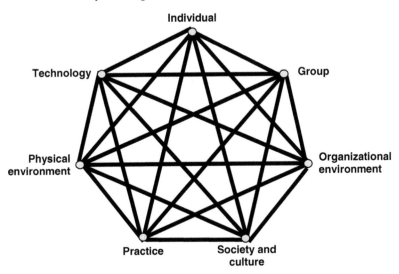

Figure 1.11 The links between all the elements in the sociotechnical model for the boat drill.

- The practice [practice] is probably shaped by the procedures and check-list [organizational environment] for boat drills on board the vessel, and the design of the equipment and boat [technology].
- The organization is probably setting standards [organizational environment] for purchase, use, and maintenance of the equipment and the boat [technology].
- The boat drill is a demand from authorities by rules and regulations [society and culture].
- The officer [individual] and the crew [group] are aware of these rules and regulations, which are also implemented by the ferry company [organizational environment].
- The practice is affected by these rules:
  - Authorities [society and culture] set up rules for the equipment and the boat [technology].
  - The physical environment sets limitations for the boat drill. In this case the weather conditions are good; the ship is in harbor and not rolling or pitching.
  - Both officer [individual] and crew [group] are aware of weather limitations [physical environment] in relation to boat drills.
  - The organization has probably set up rules for safe performance of boat drills [organizational environment].
  - There is attention from authorities that boat drills are performed in a safe manner [society and culture].

Recent accidents during boat drills could draw attention to possible dangers including a hazardous physical environment. The practice reflects the possible restrictions from weather [physical environment]: The drill is performed while the ship is in harbor. Weather [physical environment] can affect the performance of the technology during the drill (long exposure to moisture and salt can cause rust and thereby result in system malfunction).

Analyzing the boat drill in this way creates a situation where all of the elements within the sociotechnical model come or could come into play. However, one particular element deserves special attention—the physical environment. The absence of bad weather during the boat drill is influencing all other elements in the boat in a positive way. We could say that the main prerequisite for the boat drill is an acceptable physical environment (such as good weather conditions).

One final example is shown in Figure 1.12. In this case the crewmember is wearing hearing protection while working in a noisy environment. The sociotechnical system for this situation is illustrated in Figure 1.13. The influencing relationship between the physical environment and technology is also highlighted here, which is particularly important for this specific situation. Due to noise and hearing protection the officer's ability to hear audible alarms, radio calls, and so forth is strongly restricted. This could be an important observation for the design of the control panel or the organiza-

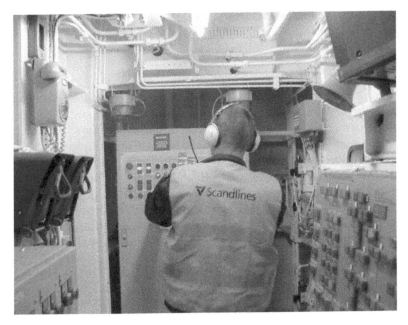

Figure 1.12 The officer is controlling the bow ramp and port of the ferry. We can see he is wearing hearing protection. The room is very noisy (physical environment).

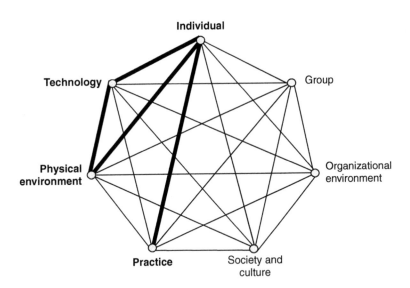

Figure 1.13 The crewmember (individual) is using the controls (technology) to close the ramp and bow port of the ferry. He is doing it in conformity with how this is usually done (practice). The place where he performs the task is very noisy (physical environment) and he is wearing hearing protection.

tion of the work (e.g., procedures for communication with the bridge about closure of bow doors).

1.6   Conclusion

The examples provided above demonstrate how the sociotechnical system model can be used in the analysis of normal situations on board ships. In some cases there might be overlapping elements or more than one system involved in the analyses (e.g., one for each vessel in the case of multiple vessels).

The usefulness of the sociotechnical model lies in the fact that it captures most of the human factors elements that form part of the maritime system. The sociotechnical system can—as a model, framework, or analytical tool— be used proactively in, for example, formulation of procedures, design of work processes, design of technology and equipment, training and education of personnel, or in risk analyses and safety assessments. Henceforth, from time to time throughout the following chapters we shall refer to the various components and interactions that form part of this sociotechnical system model.

chapter two

Individual factors:
Psychological capabilities and limitations

2.1 *Introduction*

The individual crewmember forms part of the sociotechnical system constituting the ship. Each crewmember has certain psychological capabilities and
limitations, some of which are related to the specific person, whereas others
are of a more general character. The objective of this chapter is to give a short,
basic introduction to some of the most important psychological capabilities
and limitations (or individual factors) within a maritime context. The focus
is therefore on the individual in the sociotechnical system as illustrated in
Figure 2.1.

This chapter covers a number of topics. The first section looks at human
senses and perception. The next sections cover aspects of human information processing and decision making, and the final section focuses on

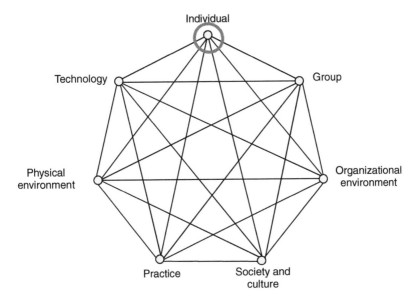

Figure 2.1 The sociotechnical system model focusing on the individual factor.

human behavior. This chapter is mainly based on cognitive psychology as it is applied in the tradition of maritime human factors. This chapter is not, and cannot be, a complete theoretical walk through the fields of cognitive psychology, simply due to the vastness of this topic. The reader is given an introduction to a number of important concepts and theories that can facilitate a deeper understanding of the psychological capabilities and limitations of the individual crewmember.

2.2   Human senses

Four human senses are significantly important in a maritime context:

- Vision
- Hearing
- Tactile senses
- Vestibular senses

2.2.1   Vision

Most of the information a crewmember uses comes from vision (although quantifying an exact percentage is almost impossible). Limitations in human vision are rather obvious; in addition, there are factors that reduce the capabilities of human vision. Vision can be impaired, although glasses and contact lenses can counteract that. Vision can be disturbed by environmental conditions such as darkness, reduced visibility, and blinding sunlight. Night vision, which we can adapt to after a while working in darkness, can be disturbed by residual light from, for example, instruments and bridge equipment. Work on the ship's bridge is characterized by extreme light conditions: from total darkness at nighttime to very bright sunlight that shines through the huge windows in the wheelhouse during daytime. Figure 2.2 and Figure 2.3 illustrate the way crew have adapted by using a blind drawn in front of a computer screen to reduce the emission of light from the screen at night.

Human vision has certain limitations. The highest level of detail and color depth is achieved in the so-called foveal vision—the point of gaze—which is only 1 degree to each side of the center of the visual field. The visual field 20 degrees on each side of the center is called the parafoveal field of vision. This corresponds to the area of visual attention and is used when looking at such things as displays or monitors. The field of vision outside the 20-degree limit is called the peripheral field of vision, and the limit of the peripheral vision is 80 degrees on each side of the center. It is not possible to see anything outside the 80-degree limit other than movements and flashing lights. The limit of the so-called binocular vision, the vision where both eyes are used together in order to perceive depth, is 60 degrees to each side of the center. Outside this 60-degree limit it is impossible to perceive depth or to see fine details.

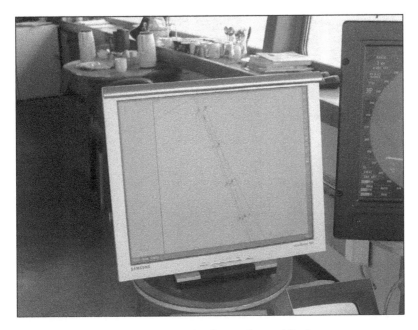

Figure 2.2   A computer screen on the bridge without a blind.

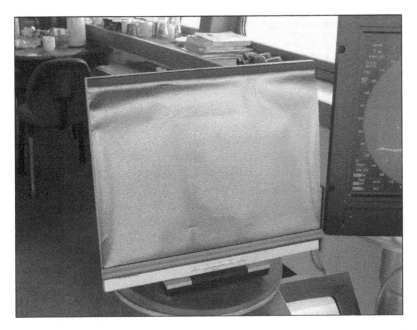

Figure 2.3   Crew adapting to a vision disturbance by placing a blind in front of the computer screen of Figure 2.2.

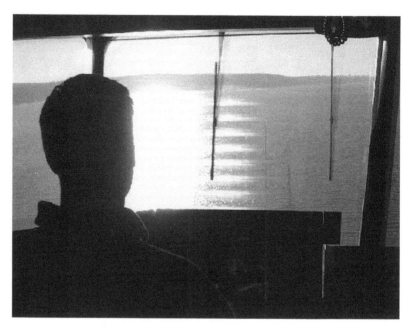

Figure 2.4 Illustration showing vision obscured by glare from natural light.

Different tools and technologies are used to overcome the problems and limitations in human vision. These range from optical devices such as glasses, contact lenses, and binoculars to sophisticated electronic equipment such as radar. Radar actually makes it possible to "see" in conditions of darkness and reduced visibility. Newer technologies, for example, those based on infrared light, are used to enhance night vision. These technologies are important in search and rescue operations, but they are also valuable when operating in waters where other vessels such as smaller fishing vessels are not using proper lights during nighttime. Blinds, sunshades, and sunglasses will help the officer working on the bridge when daylight is at its brightest. However, even using these tools, it is still very difficult to observe vessels, buoys, etc. when they are in the glare of sunlight, as illustrated in Figure 2.4.

The human vision, with its limitations, can be enhanced by the use of tools and techniques, which are important in many operations within a maritime context, especially on the bridge where exposure to extreme light and poor visibility conditions are quite frequent. The bridge and engine room layout should be designed to counteract limitations in the field of visual capability, specifically involving the parafoveal field. For example, introducing flashing lights in combination with sound signals to draw attention toward important information can assist the crew in gaining enhanced visual attention outside their normal parafoveal field (although, of course, flashing lights should be used only in moderation). The effect of lighting conditions on board ships is covered in more detail in both Chapter 5 and Chapter 6.

2.2.2   Hearing

Hearing is another human sense of great importance in maritime operations, and, like vision, it is subject to certain limitations. The two most important are the difficulties in perceiving direction of a sound signal and the disturbance from noise. These two problems are illustrated by three examples.

Example 1

A modern container vessel was approaching the harbor. When the speed was very low, an alarm signal sounded simultaneously from each of the three radar stations on the bridge. The first officer was standing right in the middle of the triangle formed by the three radar stations, and it was practically impossible for him to determine where the sound was coming from. It took him a while before he managed to locate the source and switch off all the alarms.

Example 2

A fishing trawler had five different radios mounted in a panel close to each other (Figure 2.5). All of them had one loudspeaker. The fisherman explained that they were often used together and then set to five different

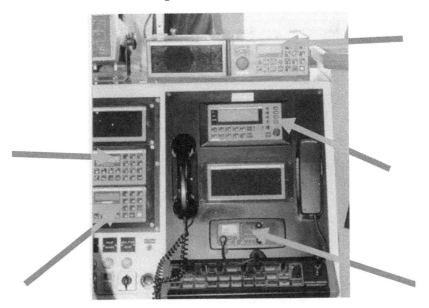

Figure 2.5   Five different radios mounted in a panel on the trawler.

channels to monitor the traffic on each of these channels. The problem occurred, as he explained, when a
call was received, and particularly when it was a very
short message; very often, it was impossible to deci-
pher from which radio, and thereby from which chan-
nel, the call was coming.

Example 3

The officer on board a ferry was working in a small
room on the car deck (Figure 2.6). The room was very
noisy and he had to wear hearing protection. The noise
and hearing protection would make it difficult for him
to communicate using the mobile radio he was holding
(the antenna was visible at his shoulder), and it would
be difficult for him to hear the phone ringing. Alarms
and sound signals in a room like this should be combined with visual signals, for example, flashing lights.

These examples illustrate how difficult it is to perceive the direction of
sound. When sound is coming from different sources at the same time, it
can almost be impossible to locate the sources, especially when positioned in
the middle of them. It is also difficult to determine the source of the sound
when loudspeakers are placed next to each other, as in the trawler example.
Knowledge about human hearing is very relevant as it can be applied to the

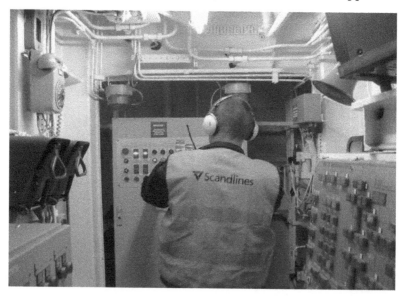

Figure 2.6 Officer wearing hearing protection equipment in a noisy part of the ferry.

design of alarms and sound signals. A better alarm signal design could have helped the officer in example 1, for example, by simply providing him with one alarm at a time, which would make it easier to perceive the direction of the sound source. Let us again look at the problem in example 3, where the focus is on maritime aids and tools related to hearing. In this case it is possible to use hearing protection specifically developed for use in noisy environments. These can have built-in radio communications and special microphones to transmit speech-generated vibrations. But these hearing aids are more expensive than standard hearing protection and mobile radios. The topic of noise (and sound) and its interaction with the individual is discussed further in Chapter 5.

2.2.3 Tactile senses

Human tactile senses are mostly relevant in relation to the design of equipment and controls. The ability to feel the differences between knobs, dials, controls, and buttons is important in situations of high stress or urgency, or when visual sense is limited. This is more applicable, for example, when using equipment while standing and turned away from it. The example below illustrates this problem further.

Example 4

The photograph shown in Figure 2.7 was taken on the bridge of a vessel and shows the control panel for the bow thrusters. Visible are two handles (with black

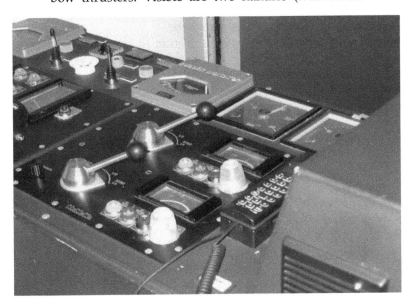

Figure 2.7   Control panel for the bow thrusters.

knobs), two dial meters, two control lights per handle (yellow and blue), and two buttons per handle (black and red). Note that the red buttons are covered with small cups usually used for liquid medicine. The cups have been placed there by the crew for the following reason: The function of the black buttons is to "take control," whereas the red buttons are emergency stops. When the officer on watch is using the thrusters in the harbor alongside a quay, he is usually standing in a position where he has his back turned to the control panel and his eyes on the window looking out. The only difference between the two buttons, which have different functionality, is their color. It is very difficult to see the color when turned away from the buttons. This had caused a problem previously when the officer of the watch pressed the wrong button (when he actually needed power from the thrusters) causing a full emergency stop at a very critical moment. To prevent this from happening again, the crew placed these cups over the emergency stop buttons. This now allows the crew to feel the difference between the black button (not covered) and the red button (covered).

Patch ups and adaptations such as the example above illustrates are very common and are seen in great numbers on almost any vessel. Figure 2.8 shows how crew used a small rope around the knob to make the tactile properties more distinct and easily recognizable.

Problems related to tactile senses are in most cases due to poor equipment design. It is obviously not possible to feel if a button is black or red or to feel the difference between three identical dial buttons. Nonetheless, the examples above illustrate that this is a common problem with the design of maritime equipment in general, and with bridge equipment in particular. Unfortunately, human factors, and the tactile senses in particular, are often not taken into account in the design of equipment within the maritime domain. In contrast, the design of controls of fighter airplanes, for example, is such that each button or dial must have significant tactile characteristics making it possible to distinguish it from others in a split second in a situation of high stress in combat—and without moving visual attention away from the action.

2.2.4   Vestibular senses

The vestibular senses are used to find the body position in space. They are involved in balance and in finding out what is up and down. They are not normally included in the syllabus of maritime human factors—and when they are

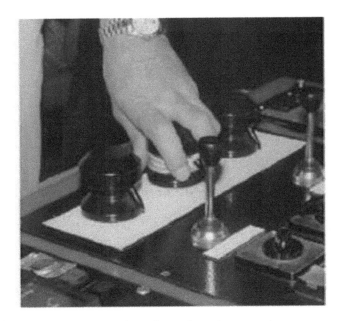

Figure 2.8 String around knob for enhanced tactile properties.

it is often in relation to motion sickness, which is examined in more detail in Chapter 5. But vestibular senses are critical for some situations. For example:

1. When the pilot, officer, or helmsman feels the rate of turn by sensing the list of the ship. The vestibular sensation of the list in this case combines and integrates with other sensory inputs. These include visual indications from the rate-of-turn instruments and gyro repeaters, visual perception of the world moving around the ship, and auditory indications from the gyro repeaters (frequency of the clicking sound).
2. When the crew feels an abnormal list indicating stability or ballasting problems.

An incident that illustrates the second example happened on board the ferry *M/V Ask* when the vessel was in harbor in Travemünde, Denmark, engaged in discharging vehicles. An auto-heeling system is used to keep the vessel upright and in balance. The system is supposed to compensate automatically when the load is moved on the vehicle decks, thereby preventing any unintended list of the vessel. When a small list occurred during discharge one time, the crew assumed that the list would soon be corrected by the system and they felt perfectly safe continuing the discharge. Unfortunately, the system erroneously did not autocorrect, and the list increased rapidly up to a point where it was critical and where damage to the stern ramp could have occurred (Figure 2.9). Fortunately, the list was noticed by

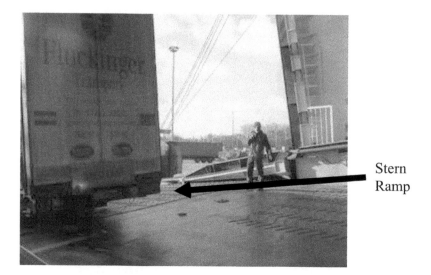

Figure 2.9 The list is increasing. When the list is critical, damage to the stern ramp could occur.

the master of the vessel from his deck office on the bridge and he immediately gave the order by radio for the crew on deck to stop unloading.

2.3   *Perception*

Our senses—seeing, hearing, and feeling—constantly give us inputs. These inputs are processed in our perceptual system. The perceptual system has, just like our senses, certain limitations and weaknesses. The fundamental function of the system is to process sensory inputs on the basis of our experience, motivations, and knowledge. If we show this text to a one-year-old child it is probably perceived as just a set of small black shapes and figures. But if we show it to an adult with English-reading skills it will be perceived as letters, words, and sentences. This mechanism is very useful because it gives us the ability to perceive more with increasing knowledge and experience. But it also has some important drawbacks: humans suffer from what is called expectation bias. This means that if we expect to recognize a certain object we will do so even if the object has changed and, perhaps, even if it is missing. For example, if an officer is looking for a certain buoy at sea he or she is actually able to observe that buoy even if the vessel is out of track and it is a different type of buoy the officer is looking at. We observe what we expect to observe.

Another concept, referred to as confirmation bias, describes a slightly different phenomenon. Confirmation bias is when we perceive only the information that can confirm our assumption and discard any information falsifying that assumption. Confirmation bias can be a serious threat to safety when the assumption is that a vessel is right on track and everything is working well. Important danger signals can be neglected simply because they do not fit with the assumption, and observations confirming the assumption will be overemphasized. There is no cure for expectation bias and confirmation bias other than awareness of the problem and a protective system of technology, crew, and procedures taking timely action when the problem occurs. The issue of awareness and technology is discussed further in Chapter 6.

Other problems are related to perception, for example, the perception of depth. Depth perception is based on experience of size and distance of objects. If we, for example, have the knowledge that a sailboat with two masts is large, we will be exposed to a visual illusion when we see a small sailboat with two masts and this is perceived as being farther away than it actually is.

Our experience is also extremely important when it comes to perception of risk. We estimate risk on the basis of our experience with accidents and incidents. If we work in an apparently safe environment we will, over time, evaluate the risk to be very low, even though the absence of accidents and incidents may be somewhat caused by "random" coincidence (what we could call luck). If an accident happens, this is added to our experience and our risk perception is adjusted to a more realistic level. The problem related to this is twofold:

1. When the perceived risk is low, our level of arousal and attention degrades slowly over time making it more difficult for us to react properly in a critical situation.
2. Low perceived risk makes us behave differently, taking more chances because we feel safe. This is further discussed in the last section of this chapter.

One way of adjusting risk perception is, from an organizational point of view, to register and disseminate information about maritime accidents and incidents. Knowledge about accidents and incidents will, even though they are not directly experienced, add to the total knowledge and experience of the mariner, thereby enabling and facilitating a more realistic risk evaluation. But only if the mariner is open minded; some people would (perhaps misled by confirmation bias) think that "this will never happen to me." Awareness about the problem will help, and risk perception is therefore often one of the subjects taught in Bridge Team Management courses.

The process of receiving information through senses and perception, as we have seen, is filled with problems and difficulties. The next section looks at what happens when the perceived information is processed further in the cognitive system.

2.4   Cognition

In the previous sections we took a closer look at human senses and perception. Information gathered through our senses via perception is processed further in what we refer to as the cognitive system. In this section we take a closer look at some theories and concepts from cognitive psychology and human factors. The selection of theories and concepts included in this book was made on the basis of their relevance in a maritime context. They also appear as part of the standard human factors repertoire of theories and concepts. The following concepts are covered:

- Memory and knowledge
- Decision making
- Attention

2.4.1   Memory and knowledge

The previous section described how we perceive using our experience and knowledge; such experience and knowledge is stored in our memory. There is a large repertoire of theories about human memory, where it is located, and how it works. We can also find a number of theories about knowledge, how it is acquired, and how it is stored in memory. Some theories are based on neuropsychological research and findings from people suffering brain damage; others are based on, for example, so-called cognitive science or information-processing paradigms. Computers have acted as inspiration for some of these theories. But, unlike computers, human memory and knowledge is distributed in the brain and not stored in one single cell or place.

Memory is normally divided in three different types:

1. Sensory memory
2. Working memory (or short-term memory)
3. Long-term memory

Sensory memory is where information gathered through our senses (visual, hearing, tactile, etc.) is stored for a very short time, usually less than one second, until enough attention is given for it to be transferred to our working memory and processed further.

Working memory is the short-term active storage of information while information is being processed or used, for example, when the Officer of the Watch (OOW) reads a bearing/distance on radar and walks to the chart table to plot the position. Working memory holds information about what activity or action we are engaged in and what the next task or activity is. It will be very difficult for us to have a normal life or go to work if our working memory is not in good shape. Severe stress can interfere with working memory, making it less robust and effective. The content in our working memory will disappear if it is not repeated or if some other efforts to retain it are not made. It is also very vulnerable to disturbances, distractions, and disruptions. Working memory has limited bandwidth; that is, it can store only a small amount of information. We therefore use, for example, notepads or voice recorders to compensate for this. An example is the built-in "replay function" in certain modern maritime VHF (very high frequency) radios. The idea is that a received message on VHF can be replayed if the listener did not manage to hear the message or if it contains more information than the listener can store in working memory (e.g., position coordinates). The replay function provides the time required to find a pencil and paper to take notes. An advantage of this is that the message can be replayed as many times as necessary. Replay functions, notepads, voice recorders, and so forth relieve the load on human working memory. It is very important to be aware that information in working memory can be destroyed immediately if the person is disturbed or disrupted. Note that disturbances are very common on ships: alarms, phone calls, radio calls, and questions from colleagues are all part of the daily routine. It is therefore very likely that the information about bearing/distance is lost if the OOW is disturbed on his or her way from the radar to the chart table. Taking notes and using checklists and other means will minimize this problem. See also "automated behavior" in the behavior section later in this chapter.

Long-term memory contains among other things our knowledge, skills, and experience. It is usually divided in what is called *declarative memory* and *procedural memory*. Declarative memory contains information and facts, and procedural memory contains our skills. In a stressful situation it is often difficult to access declarative memory, whereas procedural memory is more easily accessible. This is the reason boat and fire drills are conducted. Emergency procedures are best learned and stored as procedural memory rather than as declarative memory, because we have immediate access to procedural memory. We will not be good firefighters from classroom learning; firefighting skills should be acquired through training and drills. Another argument for drills is that memory is context dependent. This means that it is easier to remember something if we are in the same context as when it was learned. The realistic fire drill will therefore be more effective, with smoke, darkness, and so forth contributing to a context very much like a real fire, making it easier to remember the skills learned when in the real situation. Long-term memory is very robust compared with working memory, and information is often stored over long periods of time, some even for a lifetime. The amount of information stored in long-term memory is practically unlimited. Performance of long-term memory can be affected by fatigue and lack of sleep (covered in Chapter 3), in the sense that it will be more difficult to learn and store information. This will appear as "bad memory": not because the content in the memory is destroyed but because it is more difficult to store new knowledge in the memory. Mariners suffering from severe lack of sleep will often report difficulties of this sort.

2.4.2 Attention

The importance of crewmembers paying attention to tasks they are engaged in is fairly obvious. Attention is a cognitive function enabling us to focus our senses, perceptual and mental resources. We can say that the officer pays attention to the image on the radar screen, which means that he or she looks at the radar screen and processes the information from the screen mentally. It is possible to look at something without paying attention; a popular expression in Europe and Australia for this is that "the lights are on but there is nobody at home." Attention is related to all senses, not exclusively the visual sense. The ability to focus attention on a certain object or task is important: it helps us ignore irrelevant disruptions and disturbances. However, the danger with this is that we also may, in situations of extreme focus, ignore important danger signals. For example, when we try to solve problems with equipment or computers, but in the process ignore critical alarms or calls. It is therefore important that we possess the ability to distribute attention to several tasks or objects. We should be able to be properly alert even when dealing with a hardware problem. And we should be able to communicate even when we are engaged in a specific nondemanding task. Distribution of attention between several tasks is difficult when the tasks are very similar or when each single task is very complex. Individual differences will also have an influence on this. Some people find it easier to divide attention and are able to cope with more objects or tasks than are others.

Another problem related to attention is maintaining a sufficient level of attention in an extremely boring situation. The term for this is vigilance. It is not uncommon to experience boring periods at sea where nothing happens at all. No other vessels or land within visibility, no corrections of the course—just sailing a straight line for hours and hours. Similarly, in the engine control room, crew can spend long hours with no alarms, just observing and monitoring equipment. Humans are not designed for these types of situations. In fact, we are designed in a way that we automatically shut down mental processes including attention when exposed to situations like these. It is a psychological mechanism. As we do not need all these mental resources to be ready and available in these situations, we fall into a state where we appear to be awake, but in reality "there is nobody at home." It is a very dangerous situation because we can miss important sensory input and danger signals, even when we appear awake and alert. In most cases crewmembers are not directly able to notice that fellow crewmembers' level of attention is actually very low. We keep engaging in new tasks to keep our attention at an optimum level, for example, by reading news, listening to the radio, drinking coffee, or talking with colleagues. This is an effective countermeasure as long as we are still able to divide our attention and still pay heed to vital tasks when we talk, eat, drink, listen to the radio, or read the news. Chapter 3 provides more insight into the topic of mental workload, simultaneous tasks, and distractions.

2.4.3   *Situation awareness*

"In nuclear power plant incidents, operator errors relating to loss of situation awareness, flawed decision making have played a major role" (Flin 2005). We realize from this quote that "loss of *situation awareness*" has played a significant role in nuclear power plant incidents. We have no reason, however, to believe that this is not also the case in the maritime domain.

But what is situation awareness? We return to this question in a moment; let us first look at more evidence pointing at the importance of situation awareness in relation to maritime safety. In a report released by the U.S. Coast Guard in September 2006 (U.S. Coast Guard 2006) loss of situation awareness is mentioned as a risk factor in seventeen of twenty-five events in Appendix H (Safety Risk Assessment) of the report.

Although situation awareness is considered important in relation to safety it has also undergone its fair share of criticism. As Sarter and Woods (1991) wrote:

> Situation awareness has recently gained considerable attention as a performance-related psychological concept. This is especially true in the aviation domain where it is considered an essential prerequisite for the safe operation of the complex dynamic system "aircraft." There are concerns, however, that inappropriately designed automatic systems introduced to advanced flight decks may reduce situation awareness and thereby put aviation safety at risk. Situation awareness has thus become a ubiquitous phrase. Its use is most often based on an intuitive understanding; a commonly accepted definition is still missing. (p. 45)

Nine years later Dekker (2000) wrote a paper discussing similar problems in the *Journal of Transportation Human Factors*: "Although deemed an important ingredient for safe and efficient operations, crew—or joint—situation awareness remains ill defined, and results regarding its demonstration or manipulation are often unverifiable and inconclusive" (p. 49). Dekker concludes:

> Crew situation awareness has been identified as a critical factor in the effectiveness and safety of a team of humans who have to coordinate their activities with highly automated systems in the pursuit of operational goals. Yet scientific consensus on what crew situation awareness is and how to influence it appears to be far off. Many labels are used interchangeably to refer to the same basic phenomenon; results about what constitutes the phenomenon and how to measure it are fragmented, and a common definition or model is

rarely given, not even in studies that claim to demonstrate it. In this article crew situation awareness was
defined as the extent of convergence between multiple
crew members' continuously evolving assessments of
the state and future direction of a process. This definition captures various critical aspects, including the
importance of multiple subsequent assessments over
time as constituents of situation awareness and how
this evolving series of assessments allows operators to
create and share expectancies for future events. (p. 60)

From the above quotations it is evident that situation awareness is a very
important issue in relation to safety—this is also applicable within the maritime domain. Situation awareness also suffers from relevant criticism. Nonetheless, the concept of situation awareness, or lack of situation awareness,
has been used in the explanation of many maritime accidents.

Situation awareness has been studied by a number of researchers. Mica Endsley, one of the leading researchers in this field (Endsley 2002), developed the
so-called SA-model describing three successive levels of situation awareness.
A model illustrating situation awareness is shown in Figure 2.10. The model
shows three levels: perception, comprehension, and anticipation. A feedback
loop is evident between behavior and situation. This means that behavior
will change, or influence the situation (making it a new situation), and in this
regard new situation awareness on levels 1, 2, and 3 needs to be obtained.

An example illustrating situation awareness in a maritime context is the
anti-collision work on board a ship. It can be described in the following way:

1. The presence of another vessel must be detected visually or by technical means such as radar or AIS (automated identification system).
2. It must be determined if the courses will intersect; if not, there is no
   danger of collision.
3. It must be determined if there is a risk of collision, whether the two vessels will be at (almost) the same place at (almost) the same time.

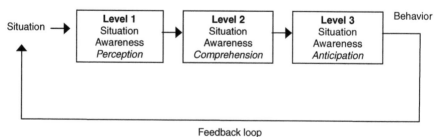

Feedback loop

Figure 2.10 The traditional way of illustrating the SA model.

4. It must be determined which ship is going to give way (according to Collision Regulations, or COLREGs).
5. Action must be taken in order to avoid collision.
6. Finally, action must be taken to ensure that the maneuver has the intended effect.

There are many ways the procedure described above can fail. The officer of the watch can fail to observe the other vessel, a wrong conclusion can be made on the risk of collision, the action taken to avoid collision can be wrong or not have the intended effect, and so forth. To illustrate the case, this process can be described in three phases using Endsley's model shown in Figure 2.10 on situation awareness:

1. Perception—Presence of other vessel must be detected (level 1)
2. Comprehension and anticipation—Will courses intersect? Any risk of collision? Which ship is going to give way? (levels 2 and 3)
3. Execution—Actions to avoid collision (behavior)
4. Feedback loop—Ensure intended effect (link between behavior and situation)

If perception or comprehension fails, we can talk about "a failure to observe the risk of collision," causing a threat to the safety of the vessel. We can see that the first step in the SA model is the perception of the situation, and that the situation could, for example, be "presence of other vessel" or "direction toward shallow water." But in a broader perspective, "what is the maritime situation and what do we need to do to describe the total situation of the ship?"

First, we should describe the progress of the vessel during the voyage: is it in open water, in restricted water, in harbor? Second, we should describe the environmental conditions, such as the amount of daylight, wind, current, visibility, and sea state. We should also describe the interaction with other vessels nearby and if a vessel is overtaking or if there is a risk of collision. Having described all relevant factors external to the vessel constituting the situation, we can proceed to the factors internal to the vessel. These include the operational mode of the vessel: what is it doing, what type of work is it performing, and which status does it have according to COLREGs? This also includes the state of awareness of the crew, the vessel, the equipment, and technology including "low technology" equipment such as charts, handbooks, and procedures, and the overall context of the vessel in the organization (e.g., if the vessel is going to be docked, if crew numbers are going to be changed or reduced, or if the schedule or route is subject to future changes). And, finally, this includes the pattern of disturbances, disruptions, and distractions (if any) at any given moment.

The above conditions can be arranged in a classification system as shown in Table 2.1. The taxonomy for classification of maritime situations described

Table 2.1   A Taxonomy for Classification of Maritime Situations

External/Internal Properties	Element in Situation	Examples
External to the vessel	The voyage	Alongside quay, harbor basin, dredged channel, restricted waters, traffic separation zone, open waters, section of route defined by procedures
	The environment	Wind, current, waves, visibility (e.g., reduced visibility as defined in COLREG), time of day
	Interaction with other vessels, vessel traffic service centers, etc.	Overtaking and risk of collision (as defined in COLREG), communication with other vessels and other stations, e.g., Vessel Traffic Services (VTS)
Internal on the vessel	The operational mode	Operational modes defined in COLREG such as underway using engine, not under command, grounded
	The state of the crew	Crew on the bridge, pilot on board, change of watch, human capabilities and limitations, attitudes, fatigue, attention
	The state of the vessel, equipment, and technology	Interaction design and usability, availability of equipment, in function, out of action, out of order, mode and settings, indoor climate on the bridge, version and update of charts, handbooks, and procedures
	The context	Long-term situation of the vessel, operational circumstances, e.g., expected change of route, reduction of personnel, major overhaul in the shipyard
	Disruptions, disturbances, distractions	Alarms, phone calls, radio calls, incoming fax, Navtex or e-mail messages, visitors on the bridge

Source: Reproduced from Koester 2007 with permission.

in the table is an attempt to come closer to the question about what the *awareness* in situation awareness is actually all about.

The idea in the situation classification system (situation taxonomy) is that the elements constitute the situation in any given case. This means that it should be possible at any given moment in the voyage of a vessel to freeze the situation completely and locate the proper descriptions for each category in the classification system. The description related to, for example, the category "interaction with other vessels" could be "no interaction what-soever." Still, this is a relevant situation, which could occur if the vessel is in the middle of the ocean. This situation taxonomy provides further insight for understanding the problems related to situation awareness in relation to the SA model in Figure 2.10. This can serve as a tool in situation-based analysis of the work on board ships, for example, in relation to design of technology, in relation to accident investigation, or in relation to development of procedures and checklists.

2.4.4 Decision making

Situation awareness is a good concept for the explanation of human behavior. Our actions are based on our perception and the processing of the perceived information, as explained in the SA model in Figure 2.10. Both perception and information processing are basic human cognitive functions. There are other theories that deal with different explanations of the cognitive processes behind human behavior, for example, theories about decision making.

We know that the mariner's decision making is important, which also relates to safety. A wrong decision could result in accidents or catastrophes. Theories about decision making primarily originated from traditional cognitive psychology, but new research has proposed an alternative paradigm different from such classical theories. The new paradigm is—as is the case with a number of other new paradigms—based on a critique of the previous theories. This critique originates from the fact that many traditional decision-making theories were based on laboratory experiments, where U.S. college students dealt with artificial problems and situations in an experimental setting. Examples of such traditional decision-making theories are as follows:

- Mental accounting
- Multi-Attribute Utility Theory (MAUT)
- Elimination by Aspects (EBA)
- Satisficing

The main criticism of these theories is that they have little ecological validity. This means that the theories convey very well how a person would make decisions in an artificial experimental setting, but little about how decisions are made in real-life situations, for example, on the bridge or in the engine room. It is quite possible that we use different strategies for decision making in the laboratory and in the field. New decision-making theories, according to the new paradigm, are therefore based on observations of decision making in natural settings rather than laboratory experiments. This paradigm is called Naturalistic Decision Making (NDM). Klein (1998) developed this theory about decision making based on observations of firefighters in the field. Klein is worth mentioning here because his theory is based on observations from a safety critical domain. This can therefore be easily applicable within the maritime domain.

NDM can, according to Klein, be characterized in the following ways:

- Many factors involved
- High risk
- Time pressure
- Dynamic problems changing over time
- Doubt about goals
- Shift in priorities
- Complex problems
- Insufficient information
- General doubt and uncertainty

The above factors of the NDM model led to another theory referred to as the Recognition-Primed Decision Model (RPD) also developed by Klein. The model maintains that in most cases decisions are made without the need to devise options, and are based on recognized situations (Klein 1998). The idea behind the RPD model is that when we are in certain situations where a decision needs to be made we try to match the situation with similar past situations experienced (from that, "recognition-primed," we recognize the situation and this will prime our decision). Our decision will then be based on previous decisions made in similar situations experienced in the past. An important point in the model is that we use "mental simulation" to antici- pate and consider the consequences of the decision. Will it also work in this perhaps slightly different case? The RPD-model can be used to understand decisions in the maritime domain and to point at the risks of failure. It is, for example, highly important that the situation is observed and perceived cor- rectly; situation awareness must be correct. Otherwise the rest of the steps in the process (decision, mental simulation, and action) will be based on a faulty foundation. Both the SA model and the RPD model can be used in explanations of human behavior. Chapter 8 looks at methods that arose from the RPD model, such as the Critical Decision Method, which are useful in collecting data on decision-making behavior for further analyses in a mari- time context.

The next section deals with other issues relating to human actions and behavior including automated behavior and risk-taking behavior.

2.5   Behavior

In previous sections we have seen how human behavior can be explained as the result of such cognitive processes as situation awareness and decision making. Now it is time to look at some issues related to human behavior and relevant in the maritime domain. This section covers the following topics:

- Skill-, rule-, and knowledge-based behavior
- Automated behavior
- Risk-taking behavior

Rasmussen (1981) proposed three levels of human behavior that relate to decreasing familiarity with the environment, thus requiring increased attention and conscious effort. There are three levels of behavior in his model:

- Skill-based behavior
- Rule-based behavior
- Knowledge-based behavior

These levels encompass most of the behavioral aspects encountered in human performance. A description of each level is provided below.

2.5.1   Skill-based behavior

This behavior mode is where most humans feel comfortable performing and actually spend most of their time in (about 80 percent). It occurs when our skills are well mastered and where most of our actions are reflex. This means the allocation of mental resources is minimal and active allocation of resources (attention) to other activities becomes possible. Driving a car is a very good example. When driving a manual car, the handling of clutch, brakes, gear, and accelerator is at the skill-based level, and we can use our attention and mental resources to watch the traffic, find our way, or perhaps even listen to the radio or have conversations with passengers in the car or on a mobile (cell) phone. Skill-based behavior is a desirable behavior mode, but it is very sensitive to routine errors. Another problem is that due to the low level of attention required to perform the task we often have no memory about the action performed. For example, when we leave our house and lock the door. Locking the door is an automated behavior; we do not pay attention while doing so, and it is therefore difficult afterward to say if we actually remembered to lock the door or not.

2.5.2   Rule-based behavior

While in this behavior mode we follow a set of formal or informal rules and procedures. This occurs when still acquiring our skill and expertise and is normal in training situations. This mode consumes a lot of mental resources leaving little room to pay attention to anything other than what we are focused on. Pitfalls in this behavior mode are work overload and making rule-based mistakes, which include errors based on a failure to apply the correct intention, or in applying the wrong rules. Mode errors using equipment in maneuvers is a typical example: the officer believes the system is set to one mode and operates it correctly according to this mode, but it is in fact set to another mode, and the operation fails. The officer is using rules for operation in the mode to which he thinks the system is set.

2.5.3   Knowledge-based behavior

This is the behavior mode where either we do not have the required knowledge or rules to apply or we have the knowledge but cannot easily recover it from our long-term memory. Finding ourselves in this mode is rare, but sometimes we are forced into it when faced with a precise situation with which we have no similar experience.

2.5.4   Automated behavior

The concept of automated behavior is often used to describe what Rasmussen calls skill-based behavior. Automated behavior is absolutely necessary to perform almost any job including tasks at sea. We need to be able to perform certain basic tasks at an automated level without using mental resources. The problem occurs when automated behavior is combined with, for example, wrong situation awareness or expectation bias: if we act automatically, based on false assumptions or on the basis of false information, there is a risk that this action could be a threat to safety. An example could be the automated reaction to what normally appears to be a false alarm: the alarm is reset when it sounds. Automated behavior, as necessary as it is, could under certain conditions compromise safety.

2.5.5   Risk-taking behavior

Another behavior compromising safety is risk-taking behavior (taking chances). Taking risks and taking chances can sometimes be well considered and well calculated, where the benefits of the actions are judged to be larger than the risk taken. Examples of benefits:

- Saving time
- Keeping schedule
- Saving fuel or money
- Keeping operation with less resources
- Making the work more cost effective

Risk-taking behavior often occurs as a result of organizational or commercial pressures. Our general perception of risk also plays a role here. We estimate risk, as indicated earlier in this chapter, based on our experience with accidents and incidents. If we work in an apparently safe environment we will, over time, evaluate the risk to be very low. We will therefore tend to take more chances and our behavior becomes more and more risky. Every time we take a chance that results in a successful outcome, we tend to add this to our experience. The result is that the next time we may behave in a slightly riskier way.

2.6   Conclusion

The objective of this chapter has been to give a short, basic introduction of some of the most important psychological individual capabilities and limitations within a maritime context. The major topics covered were human senses and perception, cognition, and behavior. Specific problems dealing with different human senses and perception were considered. An example is expectation bias, which makes us perceive what we expect to perceive rather than what we actually see. The section about human cognition has introduced concepts and models of attention, situation awareness, and decision making. This chapter has also covered the different types of memory and knowledge and specific problems related to these. Finally, we have covered human behavior, which introduced Rasmussen's theory about the three levels of human behavior and the concepts of automated behavior and risk-taking behavior. The relevance of this in a maritime context is illustrated throughout with the use of examples.

The human in the sociotechnical system—the individual mariner—has certain capabilities and limitations. Perhaps the focus has been more on the limitations and to a lesser degree on capabilities. This is because limitations are often the critical points that need to be considered when it comes to maritime safety. A general awareness of, and focus on, the perceptual and cognitive limitations as they are presented in this chapter can therefore contribute to an overall improvement in maritime safety.

chapter three

Individual–task interaction factors

3.1 Introduction

The approach taken throughout this book is to examine, as indicated in the sociotechnical system model, all the human-related elements in the maritime system and their interactions, and to assess their influence on operational efficiency and performance, as well as on operator safety, comfort, and well-being. This chapter focuses on the interaction between individual maritime operators and the tasks they are performing. This includes the individual factors as illustrated in Figure 3.1 (which is a continuation of Chapter 2), and also interactions between the individual and some of the other nodes within the sociotechnical network model (e.g., some aspects of the organizational environment not highlighted in Figure 3.1).

Many tasks in the maritime environment involve several abilities, some already described in Chapter 2, such as human senses, perception, situation

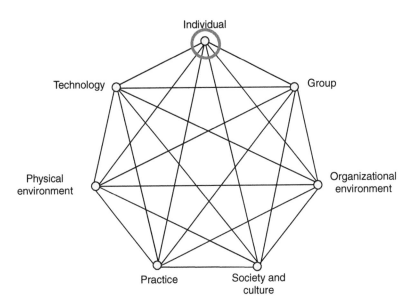

Figure 3.1 The sociotechnical system model showing the individual factor in focus.

awareness, and decision making. Other abilities include physical strength and motor skills. Often these are coordinated under stressful, tiring, and distracting conditions. These abilities are not constant; they are modified by many factors: by personal factors such as age, gender, personality, and level of maritime experience; by transient forms of impairment induced by fatigue, alcohol, or drugs; and by more permanent forms of impairment brought about by neuropsychological, medical, or musculoskeletal disorders. Particularly important here is the concept of performance-shaping factors. As the words suggest, these are features that influence how well a task is performed by an operator, positively or negatively. In this chapter we look at several key maritime performance-shaping factors, including work–rest cycles, mental and physical workload, stress, and illnesses.

3.2   Work, rest, and work–rest cycles

Most maritime environments are characterized by long and irregular working hours; hence the amount of work that crewmembers have to perform, as well as the amount of rest that they are able to take, is often not optimal. A key performance-shaping factor is the fatigue level of an individual operator. As much as possible, the crew's physiological characteristics should be accounted for in the design of the physical and organizational environment on a ship. However, as we will see below, this can be extremely difficult in the case of maritime occupational fatigue.

3.2.1   Occupational fatigue

In one sense we all know what fatigue is, and what it means to be fatigued. However, a distinction that we do not generally think about (but is accepted by most researchers in the area) is between *muscular* and *general* fatigue. Muscular fatigue comes from heavy physical work and is localized in overstressed muscles. Of most concern to us in maritime human factors is general fatigue. General fatigue can be viewed as an accumulation of all of the stresses of the day (including the duration and intensity of physical and mental work, time of day the work is performed, and the amount of prior sleep that an operator has received) and these factors need to be balanced by recuperation.

3.2.1.1   Example: fatigue in watchkeeping
Some of the main causes of operator fatigue are long working hours, sleep loss, and time of day at which work takes place. Looking at the last factor (time of day), Figure 3.2 shows a typical example of the number of errors/accidents that may be made at different times of the day by a hypothetical group of ship watchkeepers (shown by the solid line). When operators are seriously deprived of sleep, the number of errors and accidents may rise further. The broken line in the figure shows an indication of this pattern, where there is a far higher risk of accidents in the "danger" period of midnight to 6

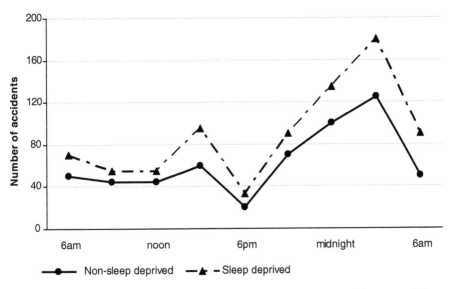

Figure 3.2   Typical example of the number of error/accidents as a function of time of the day (the solid line illustrates non-sleep-deprived operators, and the broken line illustrates severely sleep deprived operators).

a.m. (and to a lesser extent the post-lunch dip in the middle of the afternoon). In both lines in the figure it can be seen that the highest number of errors occurs between midnight and 6 a.m. (also there is a small rise in the middle of the afternoon). These kinds of error rates/performance decrements are found in many maritime jobs.

Operator fatigue is not directly measurable. Instead, indicators of fatigue are employed (e.g., subjective ratings or operator performance measures); however, these are often difficult or impossible to identify following an acci- dent. As such, quantifying the exact number of maritime accidents/incidents that involve some kind of operator fatigue as a causal factor is extremely dif- ficult. This is partly due to the accident/incident reporting systems used, and partly due to the nature of operator fatigue. Because of the difficulties in iden- tifying whether fatigue caused an accident, it is hard to estimate the contribu- tion that fatigue makes to them. In the road transport environment literature, figures of up to twenty percent of all fatal crashes involving fatigue as a main contributory factor are not uncommon. In the maritime environment where quantifications have been made, they often indicate that less than ten percent of accidents have fatigue as a causal factor, although almost certainly this is an underestimate. However, recent work in this area suggests an increase to twenty percent in these estimates. In general, however, conducting in- depth studies of accidents often finds operator fatigue somehow involved. An example of fatigue involvement in a maritime accident is the collision involving the ship *Irving Forest* with the oil rig *Gamoar Labrador* in the North

Sea in 1998. In that case, the officer of the watch dozed off because he had not slept for several days prior to the accident (due to high workload).

Looking at time on task, four hours continuously on a single task that requires high levels of concentration (e.g., monitoring navigation systems) can increase errors and incidents. Such errors might be "micro events," such as not responding to a communication. These are often more marked after seven to eight hours on shift (especially when an operator had an insufficient amount of preceding sleep). Therefore, as we will see below, planning correct working periods and breaks is essential.

Where appropriate, two strategies for combating fatigue include short naps and coffee. However, caffeine in the coffee, when used incorrectly to excess can cause both a dependency and a tolerance to develop, and can also modify sleep patterns. Techniques such as fresh air, communicating with colleagues, or stretching are not usually effective for more than a few minutes. The best solution is to obtain proper (i.e., good quality) sleep. Of course, it must be noted that on board many ships, obtaining good quality sleep can be difficult, owing to the physical environment such as noise, suboptimal sleeping areas (e.g., the quality of bedding), and ship motion. The physical environment is covered in more detail in Chapter 5.

One important issue is that once in a fatigued state, individuals find it difficult to estimate their own abilities to perform a task. Most operators are aware of the precursors of fatigue (e.g., yawning, stretching, etc.), so ideally must stop work at that point if the task is safety critical. Nobody is immune from fatigue, but sometimes the culture on a ship is for operators to deny they are fatigued until long after the symptoms have manifested (e.g., by dozing off or making frequent lapses) (Cantwell 1997). Also, in the real world of shipping, work cannot easily be simply stopped: it may not be practical, or may not be permitted. Although, with the increasing use of more "enlightened" management techniques (e.g., bridge/crew resource management discussed in more detail in Chapter 7), an operator is more encouraged to report fatigue.

Preventing fatigue from occurring in the first place (through better-designed shift schedules, fatigue management programs, etc.) is, of course, a better way to control the risk. Recently, some commercial shipping companies have introduced systematic fatigue management programs that:

1. inform workers, schedulers, and managers of the dangers of fatigue
2. encourage operators to stop if feeling sleepy
3. provide better information about sleep hygiene
4. require medical examinations (e.g., to detect sleep disorders)
5. require comprehensive records/audits

In addition, the International Maritime Organization (IMO Circ. 1014, 2001) has produced guidelines in this regard intended to inform relevant parties involved in ship safety on the nature of fatigue, its causes, and preventive measures.

3.2.2 Prolonged working hours

The number of hours worked by many maritime operators has generally been reduced over the last 100 years. However, there is a fairly widespread acceptance (by the research community at least) that long hours are a major cause of both operator fatigue and stress, and so contribute to errors, incidents, and accidents at sea. With the increased pressures of decreased crewing and commercial competition, many maritime operators still work in excess of sixty hours per week, and working ninety hours per week is not uncommon (although, of course, with large individual variations). As an example of a maritime accident due to excessive hours worked, the 1987 disaster of the capsize of passenger ferry the *Herald of Free Enterprise* was partly due to the ferry sailing with her bow doors open because the assistant bosun had fallen asleep: he had been on duty for twenty-four hours prior to dozing off. This accident is discussed further in Chapter 7.

In the industrial environment, many studies have found that increasing the length of the working day does not increase output—for example, increasing the working hours from eight to ten for a heavy manual job may even reduce overall daily output, as workers tend to "pace" themselves in longer working days. But this is, of course, not true for machine-paced work (i.e., many jobs on a ship), where it is impossible to ease up, so instead greater fatigue results. Likewise, although the evidence is not conclusive, shift durations of more than eight hours tend to increase the risk of errors and incidents. However, although limiting shift length may be physiologically optimal, it needs to be balanced against practicalities: tasks need to be performed on ships, crew have less opportunities for leisure activities compared to when on shore, and pay is often higher for longer shifts. Also, in these days of increased automation and de-crewing, operators may feel compelled to work longer hours.

Regulating hours worked is theoretically possible, but in the maritime environment (similar to the road environment) it is often impractical, inflexible, and unworkable. Some regulations do exist, such as the International Convention on Standards of Training, Certification and Watchkeeping (STCW) for Seafarers, which lays down minimum rest periods. However, aside from the issue that operators often volunteer (or feel obliged) to undertake additional periods of work, the regulations for time off duty might not correspond with the operator's circadian cycle (so making sleep more difficult) and they might hinder certain critical tasks (e.g., emergency drills) that must take place on board ships. As such, prescriptive hours of work are frequently not ideal, and more flexible alternatives (such as fatigue management) are often preferable.

3.2.3 Rest breaks

It is consistently found that rest breaks in shifts are very necessary—often they can actually increase daily output, despite slightly fewer hours "worked." There are different types of breaks and pauses, such as prescribed ones (e.g., an operator is relieved of duties for a twenty-minute lunch break), or more implicit breaks (e.g., an operator just stops or does something different, or a break due to the nature of the work such as waiting for a colleague to complete a task).

As Kroemer and Grandjean (1997) note, pauses and breaks can be especially good for:

- Heavy work (so as not to exceed daily physiological capacity for work, e.g., in terms of energy expenditure, a couple of fifteen- to thirty-minute breaks in an eight-hour shift on a ship are sometimes recommended)
- Social contacts (when an operator is working in "isolation")
- Training (so a new maritime operator has time to reflect on techniques just learned, a break of thirty minutes or more can be useful)
- Extreme machine-paced work (e.g., in the engine room, especially for the older workers, who often work slightly more slowly)
- Close visual work (e.g., to prevent temporary myopia/eyestrain among users of navigation devices, a short break looking away from the screen can help)
- Heat (to allow the body to cool down)
- Mental work (which benefits from regular short breaks, even if only five minutes per hour)

Rest between shifts is also vitally important. Adapting to varying shift patterns is often difficult, and cumulative effects of sleep loss can result in chronic fatigue (the longer an individual is at sea the worse the fatigue becomes). Such chronic fatigue can lead to deteriorations both in performance and health in the longer term. Far more than just a night or two of good quality sleep is required to recover from this.

3.2.4   Nightwork, shiftwork, and the circadian rhythm

As we all know, nightwork and shiftwork are indispensable on most ships; often it is economically essential to run a twenty-four-hour operation. Humans are naturally inclined to sleep at night (when it gets dark) and be active (work/play) during the day (when the sun rises). Many bodily functions fluctuate in a twenty-four-hour cycle called the circadian rhythm; these include temperature, digestion, and blood pressure. These bodily functions usually peak during daylight hours and are lowest at night and in the early morning hours. This trend is also associated with alertness levels. Within this context, sleep is the most important influence on the circadian rhythm.

Most people need six to eight hours sleep per night for health and well-being. Often the daytime sleep of ship-based nightworkers is of poor quality (especially when taken in noisy and cramped conditions), so has less recovery value. It is very difficult to alter circadian rhythms completely; often several weeks are needed to do this, so where they are needed, quick rotation maritime shifts are now often recommended. However, where fixed night schedules are likely, then adaptation to them is possible, especially if the operator is helped to re-synchronize by means of meals, exercise, social interaction, and light. Such adaptation can help improve the operator's health, job satisfaction, and mood. However, the demands on shipping often limit the ability to have such fixed schedules (e.g., when in port, during training, or during emergencies).

As shown in Figure 3.2, most studies have found that more work errors are likely to occur at night, that is, incidents and accidents. A standard maritime three-watch rotation can be a particular problem, with the 12 to 4 a.m. shift especially prone to problems when an operator often needs to fight to stay awake. As much as possible, where dangerous or demanding tasks need to be performed (e.g., loading), they should be done when personnel are most likely to be alert (Cantwell 1997). However, this of course can be difficult to achieve.

Nightwork can cause many health problems, such as stomach troubles, sleep problems, ulcers, and heart problems. It is estimated that two thirds of all nightshift workers experience some health complaints at some time due to their working hours (Kroemer and Grandjean 1997). Because of this, some operators in the maritime environment leave the industry.

Nightshift work can also cause social problems: less family time, little social contacts, less opportunity for clubs or social groups. The world often seems made for the 9–5ers, so shiftworkers sometimes feel on the edge of society. This, of course, is worsened for ship-based workers. Further, night-shifts are often worse for older people because they are less able to cope and less able to recover from the physiological, psychological, and physical stresses that such shiftwork brings.

Of the rest, many are "positive choice" maritime shiftworkers (i.e., they enjoy such work, and have fewer health complaints). Some positive aspects of shiftwork/nightwork can include less strict supervision/more autonomy, better pay, and sometimes more leisure time. But, overall, the drawbacks still predominate for many people.

Where shiftwork (especially nights) is needed on ships, a few recommendations (adapted from Kroemer and Grandjean, 1997) are:

- Have short shift rotations.
- Where legally possible, only use operators aged between twenty-five and fifty for shift/night work.
- Only employ healthy, emotionally stable workers.
- Avoid continuous nightwork; have at least twenty-four hours break after working a series of nights (especially if two or more nights are in the series).
- Plan some free weekends into the shift schedules.
- Ensure adequate break(s) per shift for nourishment and short rest.

Of course, some of these recommendations are not practical in every situation, but they do provide some guidance about what is best practice.

3.3   *Mental workload*

Switching the focus now, in maritime operations many manual handling tasks are still carried out, such as loading and maintenance. As such, physical workload will be considered in the next section. However, in modern shipping (with its emphasis on complex systems, automation, and decreased staffing) workload of a more cognitive or perceptual nature is a key issue. Therefore a major performance-shaping factor is mental workload. Mental workload can be defined as the amount of mental effort that is required by an operator in order to perform a task or tasks. As maritime tasks become more complex, the required mental workload generally increases.

Performance is generally best at *intermediate* levels of mental workload. If a task is too hard, obviously performance suffers; on the other hand, if a task is too easy, arousal/alertness may drop, and again performance will suffer.

3.3.1   *Workload and capacity*

Mental workload is an important issue to consider when assessing the demand placed on an operator by changes in the maritime task. The task may change because the technology has changed (new navigation or communication devices are introduced), the environment has changed (different shipping routes or working with a new company), or other tasks need to be carried out at the same time, such as speaking on a handheld radio.

Mental workload in maritime operations can vary due a large number of factors:

- the time allocated to complete a task (usually shorter periods of time allocated lead to a higher workload)
- the number of tasks performed (sometimes simultaneously)
- the difficulty of tasks
- the required level of accuracy/proficiency
- individual factors: skill, intelligence, stress, personality
- ship environmental factors: heat, noise

Mental workload assessment is further explored in Chapter 8, and how it relates to work with new ship technologies is further explored in Chapter 6.

Mental workload can therefore be viewed as an interaction among the task, the environment, and the person. Operators under high workload can compensate by increasing effort or reducing task performance. In some maritime tasks (such as routine maintenance) there are ways to reduce task load (e.g., by slowing down); however, it is more difficult to reduce task load for the majority of maritime tasks (e.g., watchkeeping or navigation).

3.3.2 Simultaneous tasks and distraction

Many maritime tasks need to occur simultaneously. For example, in the bridge an operator may be required to watch parameters on several displays, while also communicating with the engine room. Undertaking this job does not always take place in ideal conditions, in which a well-rested, well-trained, and well-behaving individual interacts with a simple, undemanding task. One issue that can make performance sub-optimal is distraction, both from within the ship and within the environment (especially when entering port). Distraction occurs when a triggering event induces an attentional shift away from the task. In the road environment, driver distraction is viewed as a critical issue, with distraction coming from many sources both inside the vehicle (e.g., a mobile phone) and in the general highway environment (e.g., roadside billboards). In the maritime environment there is generally a different set of distractions possible; nonetheless, minimizing them is still a key issue. It should be noted that the distractions are sometimes voluntary. For example, in 2000 the Greek ferry *Express Samina* struck a reef with the result that eighty passengers lost their lives; it was alleged that some of the crew were watching TV at the time. The number of possible distractions on board ships is large, so producing a definitive list to help minimize them is difficult. However, some aspects to consider are:

- When new equipment is introduced (e.g., new communication devices) how can it be integrated with existing tasks, and how does it alter existing tasks?
- The design of the operator's job (e.g., regularly changing the tasks being performed). This can help prevent underload (and the tendency for an operator to become distracted by talking to colleagues) or through "cognitive distraction" (e.g., thinking about financial issues or the spouse at home).
- Designing the environment to minimize distraction (e.g., by moving low-level machinery warning indicators away from high-level navigation warnings).

3.4 Physical workload

The focus in this book is largely on cognitive, organizational, social, and environmental factors. Despite this, physical factors are still an issue on many ships, and understanding the physical limitations and functions that affect maritime operators' lives is critical if they are to perform some tasks safely, comfortably, and successfully. As such, we briefly consider physical workload. This section starts at a fundamental level and covers some basic aspects of physical ergonomics. Then it briefly examines designing for physical work on ships.

3.4.1   *Muscular work*

Humans are able to move because of a widely distributed system of muscles, which make up about forty percent of the total body weight of an individual. The most important characteristic of a muscle is its ability to shrink to half its normal length—this is called muscular contraction. Muscle contraction involves the transformation of chemical into mechanical energy. Glucose and oxygen, the muscle's reserves of chemical energy, are only stored in small amounts in the muscle itself. Therefore both must be continuously transported to the muscles by the blood. So it is the blood supply that is the limiting factor in the efficiency of the muscular machinery. During physical work, blood is delivered around the body through an increased heart rate and an enlargement of the blood vessels that lead to the muscles.

In addition to the work produced, the muscles also produce heat. This is made up of three forms: resting heat production, initial heat (due to contraction of the muscle), and recovery heat (after contraction has finished for up to thirty minutes). For example, when maritime operators are undertaking physical activity (such as vigorous equipment maintenance work), they will usually feel warmer both during and immediately after this physical exercise than before they started.

3.4.2   *Dynamic and static muscular effort*

In terms of how physical work is performed, there are two kinds of muscular effort: dynamic (rhythmic) and static (postural). Dynamic effort is characterized by rhythmic alternation of contraction and extension, tension and relaxation. Examples of this might include walking or turning a handle. Static effort is characterized by a prolonged state of contraction of the muscles, like standing still. During static effort the blood vessels are compressed by the internal pressure of the muscle tissue, so blood cannot flow through the muscle.

During dynamic effort the muscle acts as a pump in the vascular system—compression squeezes blood out of the muscle and relaxation allows it back in again. Thus, blood and muscle waste products flow freely into and out of the muscle. By contrast, a muscle performing heavy static work receives very little fuel (sugars or oxygen), so has to rely on its own reserves. In addition, waste products (e.g., lactic acid) accumulate and produce the pain of muscular fatigue. Therefore, static muscular effort above fifteen percent of its maximum cannot be maintained for long periods and should be avoided as much as possible, and this should be considered when designing tasks and equipment (e.g., the need to grasp rope for prolonged periods).

It should also be borne in mind that the maximum force a muscle or group of muscles is capable of depends on two factors:

- Age: Peak strength is usually reached between the ages of twenty-five to thirty-five. Older operators of age fifty to sixty produce on average 75 to 85 percent as much muscular strength as their younger counterparts.
- Sex: Women have narrower muscles so on average produce 30 percent less strength than men.

The implication of this is that older crew, or those with more female members, may theoretically require additional support in some manual handling situations compared with their younger (or male) counterparts; however, the benefits of a more mixed and experienced crew will usually outweigh this in other maritime tasks. Other factors include an individual's constitution, training, and momentary motivation (where often seemingly impossible feats of strength can be evidenced in some circumstances).

How physical workload can be assessed, in terms of energy expenditure or heart rate, is described in Chapter 8.

3.5 Work-related musculoskeletal disorders

It is beyond the scope of this book to go into depth about work-related musculoskeletal disorders; however, a few words about two common types of disorders/injuries help illustrate some of the physical problems on ships.

1. *Operator back injuries* can be divided into two sub-categories:
   - Sudden overload—Usually while lifting a heavy weight, or lifting a moderate weight incorrectly
   - Cumulative overload—Repeatedly pulling or lifting a weight at a problematic angle, or using an incorrect technique; such injuries can also occur due to the physical environment such as ship vibrations, discussed in Chapter 5
2. *Repetitive strain injury* is more common in industrial assembly line workers or computer keyboard users; however, these injuries are not unknown in maritime operations. Usually they are relatively discrete and localized injuries to specific anatomical structures (such as tenosynovitis of the forearm and wrist for some frequent keyboard users).

Both these types of injuries can occur on board ships, and can be very costly to both the operator and to the company (through time off work, assignment to different duties, decreased work effectiveness, or even compensation). Good risk assessment and risk management are vital to help identify risks and ultimately control such injuries.

3.6 Anthropometrics and anatomy

Anthropometry is a subject concerned with human sizes. The term anthropometry is derived from two Greek words; *anthropo(s)* meaning human and

metricos meaning measurement. The human factors professional or ergono-
mist will use anthropometric data to ensure that the machine or the environment fits the person. Examples on ship may include ensuring that door
height or bunk sizes are adequate, or that the positions of controls enable all
operators to reach them.

Early anthropometric data came from the military environment, through
measurements of soldiers, sailors, and airmen. Nowadays a large amount of
different data for different population groups exists, and new software programs, such as PeopleSize, exist to assist in applying anthropometric data.
The variety in people's body shapes and sizes can make designing for all
users difficult. One option is to make ship equipment as adjustable as possible; another is to limit the targeted population, for example, considering
only "average" sized men, or limiting the design to the 90 percent of the
population between the extremes of size.

There are several sources of physical variability among personnel on
board ships:

- Sex. Men are generally larger than women, except in chest depth, hip
  breadth, hip circumference, and thigh circumference.
- Age. People generally shrink in height as they get older, and often
  get wider.
- Ethnic background. Different ethnic groups are different heights, for
  example, Swedes and Americans are usually taller than Thais and Japanese. As such, a multinational ship's crew is likely to comprise of a
  range of sizes.

3.7 General principles of workstation design on ships

Again, it is beyond the scope of this book to cover too much information
about ship workstation design. However, such factors can be considerably
important to the individual operator (by affecting morale and motivation),
and may influence how well a task is performed. The issue of equipment
design is considered in more detail in Chapter 6, but some issues should be
addressed within workstation design on ships:

- Clearance for larger operators (e.g., bed, corridor head clearance, or
  door sizes).
- Reach for smaller users (e.g., reach zones when stacking freight).
- Static muscular effort. As discussed above, this should be avoided as
  much as possible.
- Adjustability (e.g., bench height for maintenance work). Although
  adjustability is important, it is equally important that adjustments are
  made correctly. For example, an operator may leave a bench adjusted to
  the last user (who may be of quite a different size).

- Seating. Where a task is to be performed seated, then a suitable chair should be provided. Sadly, there is no single, ideal seat for all occasions. Different tasks, people, and jobs require different seats. However, having one with appropriate support (e.g., backrests), simple adjustments, and good stability are some of the main factors.
- Visibility (e.g., matching the focal length of a display screen, i.e., the distance between a users eyes and the screen, to the likely users, especially when the probable user's are older operators).
- Component arrangement (both within a single piece of equipment, for optimal eye and hand control movements, and for different pieces of equipment required to perform a single task). For example, on the bridge, often different tasks have a separate workstation assigned to them: one for route planning/navigation functions, another for radio and communications, and another for maneuvering/traffic surveillance.

3.8 Stress

Folklore may tell us that a little stress can sometimes be a good thing; it can motivate individuals, and help them focus on a task. However, we believe that psychological stress, properly defined, is always a negative factor. Psychological stress on ships means that crewmembers may perceive tasks, environmental, and/or internal demands, as nearing the limit or exceeding their resources for managing the situation. In terms of its effects on maritime task performance, stress can make the crew focus more narrowly on a few specific aspects of their task and neglect other aspects, possibly leading to negative consequences. Also, stress can increase the likelihood that crewmembers may engage in unsafe, risky behaviors by adopting "short-cut" work methods, whereby onboard safety rules and procedures are not properly followed.

Therefore, if there is high time pressure and high stress on ships, the crew may think that taking risks is simply part of their job and that there is not always time to follow safe procedures. Shorter-term reactions to stress may include "flight or fight" (e.g., abandoning the task or confronting colleagues), increased anxiety/agitation, more arguments between crew, and increased use of alcohol or illegal drugs. In the longer term, issues such as job burnout and increased health complaints can be evident (such as digestive or cardiovascular problems).

Over the years, there have been an increasing number of studies investigating stress at sea. To take one example, Riordan, Johnson, and Thomas (1991) investigated stress among commercial fishermen. They found that the fisherman experienced more stressors than a comparison group of land-based workers: among the chief culprits were working long shifts and having responsibility for the lives of others. Having some degree of "mastery" (or control) over a situation helped to reduce stress. However, being away from family and friends was a significant stressor for fishermen (and, of course, for other maritime operators) (Riordan et al., 1991).

Stress might be an issue particularly for younger operators who are still learning many onboard tasks. It can also be a problem for older operators, who may have less ability to cope with task demands due to declining physical capabilities (e.g., strength or resistance to fatigue) and perceptual/cognitive capabilities (e.g., failing vision or impaired memory).

As a result of the individual nature of stress (which depends on how operators perceive the demands and perceive their ability to cope with such demands), it is sadly not easy to provide many general task recommendations to reduce its occurrence. It is not simply an issue of a "level" of stress for the individual in the task/environment that should not be exceeded. However, stressors like being away from one's family and friends during long periods at sea can affect most crew, and are difficult to manage. The support networks on ships are usually far from optimal; however, greater communication between crew and their supervisors or ship medical officers can help to identify risks. The use of formal safety management programs that focus on aspects such as open communication and risk assessment should be encouraged.

3.9   Illness, concerns, anxiety, and pressures

In addition to stress, other factors may negatively influence how an individual performs a task. Some of these are briefly reviewed below. First, we briefly look at physical factors, and then we examine what broadly could be classified as "psychological" factors.

3.9.1   Effect of physical illness

In many ways a ship is quite a physically enclosed environment; therefore, contagious diseases can often spread more easily than they would on dry land. Although cases of more severe diseases and illnesses on ships are somewhat fewer now than they were a few centuries ago, ships are still environments where minor illnesses can be passed on easily. This is heightened by crew coming from several different nationalities, where their immunities from different diseases are variable.

As an example, colds and influenza may be easily transmitted on a ship. Often the consequences of colds are relatively small, and some crew simply would work on while suffering from a cold. However, such a minor illness would still have an impact on task performance—especially if the operator needs to perform outdoor work in difficult environmental conditions (like operating cranes or lifting equipment), or to undertake tasks in which a high level of cognitive effort/vigilance is needed (like navigating and piloting). Likewise, many products that relieve the symptoms of colds contain alcohol or other legal drugs, so this may further reduce task performance.

Earlier in this chapter we saw how the physical environment can result in work-related injuries (e.g., back injuries and upper limb disorders). Although notions like "accident proneness" are not commonly accepted today, it is still true that injuries or accidents do not affect all operators equally. Some operators are more hardy/robust, and people have differing degrees of health consciousness. People also differ in how they perform tasks (e.g., they use different lifting techniques). As such, despite training and selection, there is variability in people's ability to withstand the demands of life at sea.

The implication of all this is that minor illnesses might be prevalent in a ship's crew at any one time, often with performance implications (to a greater or lesser extent). Equally, different operators have different health-related attitudes and behaviors, and have somewhat different tolerances to withstand different task demands. Given the often macho culture that still exists on many ships, there is a tendency just to work through such issues. Careful and systematic management of the issues would be optimal, although this is not always possible to achieve in practice by ship-based management.

3.9.2 Effect of concerns, anxiety, and pressures

In this chapter we saw how distraction may negatively affect successful task performance. As well as distraction caused by external events (e.g., conversations between crew or paying unnecessary attention to other ships nearby), operators may be subject to cognitive distraction, such as worrying about domestic/family issues, or more general worries about organizational issues and career direction.

By its very nature, a ship is a very constrained environment in which crew can be away from their families for long periods of time. Better communication technologies (such as e-mail or satellite phones) can be useful tools to reduce this emotional deprivation and can help operators cope with the stressor, at least where such communication devices are present. However, being physically away from family, friends, and shore-based support and entertainment can still be a significant challenge. As we saw within the discussion of shiftwork, often maritime shiftworkers are positive choice workers, who can in part adapt their lives successfully to more irregular hours of work; those who cannot adapt often leave for jobs that involve significantly less shiftwork. To some extent the same is true of more general adaptation to life on a ship; those operators who can successfully organize their lives around long periods of being away from a more traditional home life are those who are more likely to stay working in the industry for longer periods of time.

3.10 Alcohol

We end this chapter by considering alcohol. Temporary impairments due to alcohol or drug use can have a huge influence on crew behavior. Historically, there has been a common perception that alcohol was a problem on board ships. Alcohol-impaired maritime operators have been involved in a significant number of accidents and incidents. For example, the master of the *Exxon Valdez* was reportedly under the influence of alcohol when the ship ran aground on a reef in Alaska in 1989, which caused the world's largest environmental disaster. Sadly, the inappropriate use or abuse of alcohol still permeates some maritime environments.

The amount of alcohol in the blood is commonly measured by blood alcohol content (BAC). Most shipping organizations today have an alcohol policy, and within the International Convention on Standards of Training Certification and Watchkeeping for Seafarers (STCW) Code limits of 0.08 percent BAC now apply. In general terms, operator performance functions, such as reaction time, tracking, attention, perception, and motor skills, are all worse with higher BACs.

With greater knowledge about the effect of alcohol and more widespread testing its use is now diminishing.

3.11   Conclusion

The whole issue of how an operator's job is designed has received a large amount of attention in industries like manufacturing, but traditionally less so in the maritime environment. Concepts like autonomous work teams, job enlargement, and job enrichment have all been extensively studied in manufacturing; in the maritime industry, job rotation is often the limit of how an operator's job is varied. Job rotation involves operators being moved between different tasks; this rotation can occur within shifts or over longer time periods (e.g., one week for one type of task, and the second week for a different type of task). Job rotation within a shift is especially useful for tasks that are either very physically or cognitively challenging or where training has just taken place (where job rotation can allow an operator to reflect on what he or she has just learned).

Finally, a ship is like many other workplaces where issues like organizational pressures and the pressure to achieve have considerable effects on the individual operator. As we have seen when discussing stress, different people perceive and cope with such pressures differently. However, given the constrained ship environment where an operator usually cannot fully get away from work at the end of their shift, the effects of such pressures are usually greater than shore-based work, as, for example, Riordan et al. (1991) found for fishermen in the United States. Therefore, although we can do a great deal to help improve the ergonomics and the organizational environment on a ship, the personality of individual operators is still a major factor in helping them to cope with the pressures at sea.

In Chapter 7 we examine in more detail the interaction of organizational and individual factors; however, organizational factors are also performance-shaping factors regarding how successfully an individual can complete an individual task.

chapter four

Communication and team work

4.1 Introduction

Communication and teamwork are two of the traditional, as well as fundamental, ingredients of the syllabi of crew resource management and bridge team management courses. Optimal communication and teamwork are essential for onboard safety, as breakdowns in communication or teamwork could cause accidents. This chapter presents some important concepts and models related to communication and teamwork. Applications of the concepts and models are illustrated using different examples, primarily from the maritime domain.

The focus of this chapter is on the interaction between individual and group as illustrated in the sociotechnical system in Figure 4.1. The first part of this chapter focuses on communication and the second part on teamwork.

4.2 Communication

There are a variety of different threats to optimal communication. Verbal communication can be difficult in noisy environments, as mentioned in Chapter 5. It can also be problematic when using technical communication devices with poor sound quality (e.g., radio, mobile phone), or even due to language problems as indicated in Chapter 1. Two vessels communicating might need to use a common language—for example, English—which may not be the mother tongue of any of the parties involved. Language problems are also common on board ships with mixed nationality crews, where misunderstandings due to language problems can have fatal consequences. Let us look at some examples.

Example 1

This incident occurred on board the vessel *M/V Sally Mærsk* in June 2000 while on a voyage from Hong Kong to Long Beach, California. A repairman from Poland was suffering from back pain and fever. Due to his poor English language abilities he asked his colleague, another repairman from Poland, to be his interpreter during the medical consultation with the chief officer.

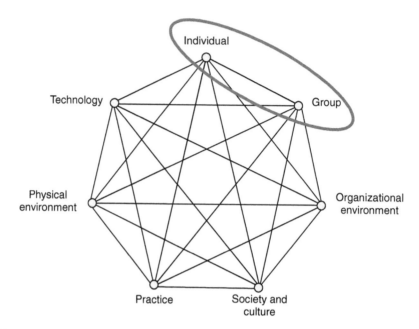

Figure 4.1 Interaction between individual and group within the sociotechnical system model.

The sick repairman had injured his back a few days before. His colleague was aware of this and assumed that the pain was caused by this injury. The sick repairman explained and asked his colleague to translate that he had pain and felt sick with fever. However, the information about the fever was somehow lost in the translation, with the chief officer now assuming that the problem was caused by the injury. The chief officer prescribed mild pain killers as the only treatment. Over the next two days the sick repairman complained to his Polish colleague about his ailments, specifically the fever which had become worse. During the last visit the sick repairman seemed to be asleep and his colleague left him without talking to him. Later that day the sick repairman was found dead. The cause of death was diagnosed as pneumonia.

Example 2

In 1966 the ferry *Skagerak* was on route between Norway and Denmark but foundered in heavy weather. The passengers and crew were all saved due to a

remarkable effort by the crew, as well as by the vessels and helicopters engaged in the search and rescue operation. The mustering of the passengers was
not done using loudspeakers. A member of the crew
knocked on every cabin door and asked passengers in
Norwegian or Danish to don their lifejackets and go to
the mustering stations as quickly as possible. A couple
of French-speaking passengers did not understand the
instructions given and assumed that the crewmember
was talking about the arrival. They therefore dressed
carefully in preparation for the presumed arrival and
went to the passenger area. There they found other passengers dressed in pajamas and lifejackets. Although
the situation can now be considered amusing—these
passengers were in fact saved—it is evident that the
problems with communications between crew and
passengers could have had fatal consequences.

Verbal communication takes time, and this is especially a problem in a critical situation. But even in everyday communication excessive time pressure
could be a problem, slowing the speed of communication; that is, increasing the time taken to get the message across, and making it less effective.
However, certain mechanisms can help counteract these problems, leading
to easier and more optimal communication:

- Multimodal communication
- Context and mutual understanding
- Closed loop communication

The next section is a walk-through of some concepts and models that can be
used in the description and analysis of different aspects of communication. We
conclude this section with a discussion about the role and power in communication, which will lead us to the second part of the chapter on teamwork.

4.2.1   *Multimodal communication*

Communication on a ship is often "multimodal." This means that many channels of communication are in use at the same time. For instance, Figure 4.2
shows crewmembers loading concrete blocks onto the deck and unshackling
lifting chains using voice and gesture communication.

The use of different channels of communication is important—especially
in a noisy environment like the one illustrated in Figure 4.2. We can easily imagine how an occupational accident could happen in Figure 4.2 if the
interaction (communication and teamwork) between the two crewmembers
breaks down. In the picture, the deckhand is swinging a hammer (shown as

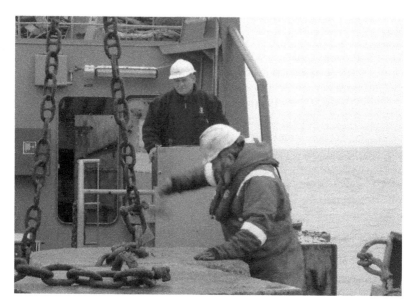

Figure 4.2 Crewmembers loading concrete blocks onto the deck using voice and gestures for communicating.

a blur in the image) to free the shackle. The crane operator needs to coordinate the lift with the crewmember working with the hammer and shackle. A serious injury can still occur if the timing is misunderstood, and the concrete block is lifted at the wrong moment (even though the hardhats offer some level of protection). In this particular situation hand signals are used as a means of communication to supplement the verbal communication (which is of limited quality due to noisy environmental conditions). It is also obvious that the two crewmembers share the same context, and that the actions performed by one of them are signals to the other. The actions have a communicative content. The shackle being dismantled is a signal to the crane operator; the concrete block settling on deck also provides a signal to start the work on the chain and shackle.

The use of gestures in communication is important. Gestures, like pointing at a radar screen, a chart, or a document, are often seen as part of the bridge communication. The pointing gesture help the parties involved in the communication to appreciate that it is "exactly this plot on the radar," "exactly this buoy in the chart," or "exactly this turning point in the voyage plan." Pointing at an object makes it a lot easier to confirm that we are talking about exactly that same object. Figure 4.3 illustrates a situation where the captain and the chief officer are discussing vessel maneuvers in front of an electronic chart screen. The ability to look and point at the same screen makes communication a lot easier, with enhancement of the quality and accuracy of communication.

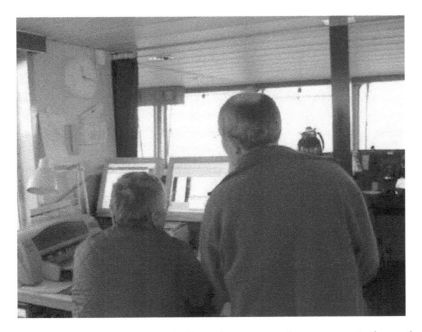

Figure 4.3 Captain and the chief officer discuss vessel maneuvers in front of an electronic chart screen.

Communication is usually more inefficient, and the risks for misunderstandings are higher, when multimodal communication is impossible or difficult, for example, when communicating over a radio or mobile phone. It is also important to note that even when multimodal communication is possible and in use, this does not in itself guarantee that communication will work flawlessly and efficiently. Hand signals, gestures, and verbal intonation can be misunderstood, even among experienced work colleagues.

4.2.2   *Context and mutual understanding*

Human communication is heavily context dependent. A major part of the meaning and understanding constructed from communication exchanges is derived from the shared knowledge and mutual context of the actors involved in the communication. A lot is necessarily left unsaid, because:

- it is part of the *shared knowledge* and skill. For example: We do not tell the helmsman how to turn the rudder when giving a rudder command and we do not explain what Vessel Traffic Services (VTS) means when sharing the content of a call from VTS; or
- it is part of the *mutual context* for all the actors involved. For example: The topics talked about in the communication are present in the environment so everybody can see or hear what is being talked about. An

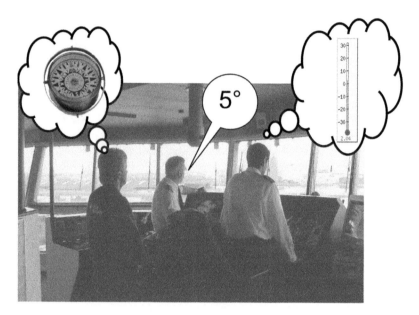

Figure 4.4 Problems with mutual misunderstanding, where "5 degrees" can be interpreted in two ways on the bridge.

example could be another ship posing a potential collision threat, with the bridge crew discussing the threat and how to avoid it.

Mutual understanding is important for normal everyday communication. But mutual understanding can easily turn into mutual misunderstanding. The example in Figure 4.4, although a bit exaggerated, illustrates the problem of mutual misunderstanding quite well. The captain giving an order of 5 degrees is understood immediately by the helmsman as 5 degrees on the compass. However, if the conversation has just been about the weather and the officer still has this context in mind the 5 degrees could be misunderstood as meaning 5 degrees Celsius, referring to the outside temperature.

The best defense against false mutual understanding is to have clear and efficient procedures for sharing routine information, such as rudder commands that are required to be repeated by the helmsman, who is also required to inform the captain when the actions have been carried out. This way of communicating is often called closed-loop communication.

4.2.3 Closed-loop communication

Closed loop communication contains three very basic steps:

1. Order or observation is spoken out loud and clear;
2. The receiver of the order or observation repeats the exact message; and

3. The sender of the message confirms that the repeated message is correct.

An example is:

1. Lookout: "Fishing vessel ahead 45 degrees to port!"
2. Officer on Watch (OOW): "Fishing vessel ahead 45 degrees to port!"
3. Lookout: "Roger!"

Or:

1. OOW: "Steady on 203!"
2. Helmsman: "Steady on 203!"
3. OOW: "Thank you!"

Apart from protecting against false mutual understanding, the strategy of closed-loop communication has some advantages: when an order or observation is spoken out loud and clear it is often heard by all persons present—this will support team situation awareness. Sometimes just as the order or observation is spoken out or when it is read back to the sender of the message it becomes clear that the message was wrong. For example: "45 degrees to port" should have been "45 degrees to starboard" or "steady on 203" should have been "steady on 302." It is often easier to realize that we have made a mistake if the mistake is spoken out loud or when we hear our own words repeated by a fellow crewmember.

4.3   *Social role and power*

As in virtually all professional work, social role and power relations in maritime operations influence the form and meaning of communication exchanges. Social roles defined by the division of labor (such as "Officer on Watch" and "helmsman") and by regulations* superimposed on the activity will influence communication. According to the Danish psychologist Knudsen (1985), two dimensions are represented in any communication: (1) The power dimension; and (2) the role symmetry dimension.

As shown in Table 4.1, the power dimension is related to how the two participants engage in communication. Are they trying to gain and demonstrate power to each other? The role symmetry dimension on the other hand is related to the formal roles of the two participants. These could be symmetric (e.g., two friends talking) or unequal (e.g., pilot and master, or master and mate).

In *power-free* and *symmetric* relations, debates and discussions are possible. This is rarely the case in bridge operations; nevertheless it may possibly

---

* The COLREGs (Collision Regulations), for example, define roles in ship-to-ship encounters, and therefore also define roles for communication such as "stand on vessel" and "give way vessel."

Table 4.1   Power and Role Symmetry Dimensions in Communication

	Symmetric Relation	Unequal Relation
Power relation	Fight, Quarrel	Interrogate, Order
Power-free relation	Debate, Discussion	Request, Suggestion

occur in teams with unclear leadership. In power-free and symmetric relations, debates and discussions are important to explore new solutions to problems if time and mental resources for this are available. However, this "democratic" ideal is not appropriate in safety-critical work, where a clear division of labor will define unequal roles for the human actors.

On board ships, the participants are to some extent unequal, in the sense that the different actors participate with their different competence and from their different assignments on board. In this regard, maritime teamwork (i.e., relations between master and officers and/or officers and ratings) is in most cases defined as a *power* and *unequal* relation (as identified in Table 4.1). Some of the communication on the bridge, or between bridge and deck or between bridge and engine room, will be in the form of short orders and confirmations following set procedures for these exchanges. This is a rational way of handling routine exchanges defined by power and social role. Orders, however, will not solve the problem in more complicated situations, such as when a pilot is on board or when resolving particular problems such as navigation, maneuvering, and engine control, and so forth. Communication in these cases should ideally take the form of requests for information, and suggestions for possible solutions, but this only occurs in power-free relations.

4.4   *Four dimensions of verbal communication*

Metze and Nystrup (1984) define four dimensions of verbal communication in a professional context. Any communication sequence (conversation, statement, order, question, answer, etc.) can be analyzed according to these four dimensions (Figure 4.5):

1. *Cognitive* (knowledge and sense, exchange of exact information) — *affective* (feelings and intuition)
2. *Expanding* (long conversation or dialogue, questions which lead to comprehensive answers) — *limiting* (closing the conversation as quickly as possible, short answers, yes/no)
3. *Confronting* (focus on problems and conflicts) — *concealing* (hiding problems and conflicts)

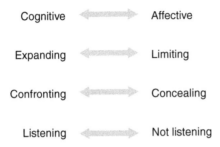

Figure 4.5 The four dimensions of verbal communication by Metze and Nystrup (1984).

4. *Listening* (paying attention to what is said and showing that by gestures or answers) — *not listening* (not paying attention, indifferent, no eye contact)

Whether communication should be expanding or limiting varies depends on the context and purpose of the communication. The command/confirm communication, which is used on the bridge, is an example of limiting communication, which, of course, is appropriate in the given situation (Pyne and Koester 2005).

The content of the communication (a specific sentence or set of sentences of verbal communication) could be characterized as being on a continuum between cognitive and affective, between expanding and limiting, and so forth. A simple example is that communication can be characterized as being more cognitive than affective, equally cognitive and affective, or more affective than cognitive. It could be hard to understand how communication could be characterized as both listening and not listening, since not listening is the negation of listening, but certain communication sequences could have both listening and nonlistening characteristics, for example:

> The helmsman is talking to the captain on the bridge. The captain is answering, replying politely saying "yes, okay, I see" (the listening element of the communication) while at the same time he looks out of the window using his binoculars (the not listening element of the communication).

Metze and Nystrup (1984) have put forward a theory about good professional communication. They indicate that it should be cognitive rather than affective, confronting rather than concealing, listening rather than not listening, and expanding or limiting according to the given context. Professional communication in the maritime domain will often deal with facts, observations, orders, and so forth. These are all in the cognitive end of the spectrum. If the communication becomes affective it is about emotions, attitudes, and so forth. This type of communication is often seen in quarrels and arguments, which should always be avoided in the maritime domain for safety reasons. Concealing communication could be very dangerous. For example, not giving important information but hiding it for some reason (e.g., fear of punishment) could cause mishaps and accidents (see the example of the KLM accident in the section Authority Gradient later in this chapter). The listening property of the maritime communication is very well demonstrated from the principles of closed-loop communication. A captain giving a rudder command to the helmsman will receive a confirmation from the helmsman indicating that he or she is listening (although, as mentioned in both Chapter 2 and Chapter 6, this does not necessarily imply understanding). The confirmation will have the form of the repetition of the command. The captain will, in order to close the loop, acknowledge this confirmation through a listening attitude, for example, answering "yes" or "ok," as illustrated in the example below.

Captain: "Starboard 10!"
Helmsman: "Starboard 10!"
Captain: "Ok!"

4.5 Transaction analysis

Metze and Nystrup's (1984) model is designed for the analyses of communication in a professional context, unlike transactional analysis, developed by the psychiatrist Eric Berne, which is designed for persons in psychotherapy (Berne 1961). The model developed by Berne is, however, now very popular and is also used in the analysis of communication in professional settings.

Berne's book *Games People Play: The Basic Handbook of Transactional Analysis*, first published in 1964, contains his main work, although he had already introduced transactional analysis in an earlier book *Transactional Analysis in Psychotherapy*, published in 1961. Transactional analysis is a method for studying interactions between individuals. It deals with three ego states referred to as: Parent, Adult, and Child. The ego states are concepts independent of the everyday meaning of the words parent, adult, and child. An ego state is defined as "a consistent pattern of feeling and experience directly related to a corresponding consistent pattern of behaviour" (Berne 1961, p. 13), with the most simple transaction occurring between two adult ego states. This is also the best type of communication in a professional context. Crossed transactions, for example, between the ego state Parent and the ego state Child, should be avoided. An example of this is an argument where communication can be characterized by talking down and reproaching. This type of communication should never occur in a professional work environment. Another example is patronizing, which should be avoided, as this can lead to humiliation and confusion. It also produces childlike behavior (talking back, teasing, etc.), because "the child" in the person spoken to is being addressed. The following example illustrates cross-communication:

Pilot (Adult ego state) to captain (Adult ego state): "Should I ask for tugs to be standby?"
Captain (Parent ego state) to pilot (Child ego state): "I have told you before that we do not need tugs! Why don't you listen to what I tell you?"

4.6 Teamwork

It is, of course, important to work together as a team within a maritime context. Maritime teams are often characterized by a formal construction based on the traditional roles of master, mate, officers, ratings, pilot, and so forth. The hierarchy is strict and formal. It is important to know the essential concepts when analyzing and discussing maritime teamwork: these are authority gradient and leadership style.

4.6.1 Authority gradient

The concept of authority gradient is used to describe the relationship between people of different rank and/or authority working together. The authority gradient is said to be low (flat) or high (steep) according to the character of the communication and interaction between two people. The authority gradient is the result of the combination of the authority of the captain/officer and the assertiveness of the mate or crew. The authority of the captain could be high and the assertiveness of the crew low. This would make the authority gradient steep. If a high authority is matched by a high assertiveness the authority gradient will appear flatter.

It is possible to distinguish between the formal authority gradient based on the ranks of the two people, for example, master ranking higher than mate, and the informal authority gradient based on personal appearance and behavior, leadership style, and communication, for example, two crewmembers of the same rank with different ages or different amounts of experience.

Probably one of the most famous accidents illustrating the danger of steep authority gradient is from aviation. It involves the collision between two commercial aircraft (a Pan Am and a KLM Boeing 747 airplane) that occurred on the runway in the Los Rodeos airport in Tenerife in 1977. The authority gradient in the cockpit of the KLM airplane was very steep. The captain (Van Zanten) of the KLM plane was one of the highest ranking officers in the organization. Even when the copilot realized that Captain Van Zanten made a mistake, he did not dare question his decision. He did, however, make one attempt, but Captain Van Zanten opened the throttle for takeoff. The copilot did not have the assertiveness to make a second attempt to prevent a disaster. The KLM airplane did not have clearance to take off because a Pan Am airplane was still on the runway. Captain Van Zanten was eager to take off and did not wait for clearance. A collision was inevitable, and the KLM airplane hit the Pan Am airplane on the runway killing most passengers on both aircraft.

Leadership style and communication are important in relation to authority gradient. Even though a high formal authority gradient is present, appropriate leadership style and communication can reduce the slope of the gradient.

Culture is important when it comes to authority gradient, as highlighted in Chapter 7. Hofstede (1997) used the concept "power-distance" to characterize the culturally dependent authority gradient. In some cultures it is highly unlikely that a rating would question decisions made by his or her superior, as illustrated in the following accident. The grounding of the Malaysian flag container ship *Bunga Teratai Satu* on the Great Barrier Reef in Australia occurred when a waypoint alteration was not made. The significant act that caused the accident, as identified by the accident investigators and which led to the missed waypoint alteration, was a telephone call made by the Pakistani mate and his wife to their family. The mate had developed a practice of asking the able seamen (AB) from Myanmar to plot the ship's position from the GPS (Global Positioning System) every hour when the ship was in open waters. As the pilot had left the ship and they were out of the compulsory protection zone, but not onto their next waypoint, the AB assumed his role and proceeded to plot this position. The position plotted was adjacent to waypoint 34 on the ship's passage plan, where the ship's course was due to be altered. In this regard, the AB had to wait for the mate to give the order to alter the ship's position. According to the AB, he kept expecting the mate to come back into the wheelhouse to alter course. But the mate did not reenter the wheelhouse for a while as he was occupied with the telephone conversation with his family in Pakistan. Only after making some coffee did the mate go over to the chart table. At this point he noticed that the AB had made a mistake in plotting the position. Frantically, he told the AB to "change to hand steering," but it was too late as shortly afterward the vessel ran aground. The AB was obviously an intelligent young person with some six years seagoing experience. He had learned to plot GPS positions but was not familiar with chart symbols or issues such as scale or time/distance estimations. He did not realize the ship was heading into danger. He continued his lookout duties assuming that the mate would appear and make the appropriate alteration in due time. Such an attitude reflects a steep authority gradient, and in their account of the accident, investigators noted that there existed a strict hierarchy between the Pakistani senior officers and the Malaysian, Indonesian, and Myanmese junior officers and crew. It was important in the national culture of the crew that the AB, although he knew that something was wrong, did not question the decisions of his superior.

It is very unlikely that this grounding would have occurred had there been a Scandinavian or Australian crew, simply because the power distance is less significant in the Nordic and Australian cultures. Low power distance helps in creating and maintaining self-directed teams, because empowerment is easier to achieve in these types of cultures. Countries with high power distance are ones where employees are seen as frequently afraid of disagreeing with their bosses. Using the Metze and Nystrup model, the communication on the bridge before the grounding of the *Bunga Teratai Satu* could be described as cognitive (about facts), limiting (command–confirm style with no room for questions from the AB), concealing (the AB concealed his awareness about the mistake made by his superior due to the cultural factors described above), but, in general, listening. Contributory causes of this accident can be found in the limiting and concealing qualities of bridge communication.

4.6.2 Leadership styles

Authority gradient is closely related to the style of leadership. Both authority gradient and style of leadership are to a wide extent defined by the characteristics of the communication. It is possible to operate within four different leadership styles:

1. Autocratic
2. Laissez-faire
3. Self-centered
4. Democratic

4.6.2.1 Autocratic leadership style

The captain (or officer) plays solo, does not pay attention to the opinions of others, does not listen (not listening according to the Metze and Nystrup model), does not share tasks or cross checks, and passes no information to the crew. The style is also often characterized by lack of planning, and the captain (or officer) is highly likely to be overloaded if a problem or critical situation occurs. The autocratic leadership style is influenced by factors such as:

- Differences in seniority and technical skills
- Tradition
- Personality: perceiving cooperation as criticism and refusing it
- A captain/officer's strong autocratic personality
- An officer/rating's weak, self-effacing character
- A captain/officer's lack of self-confidence and use of authority to conceal this

Crew reactions to the autocratic leadership style are often simply withdrawal. The result is a non-efficient bridge team where this leadership style could be a threat to safety. The master would make unsafe decisions, purely on his own accord. Nobody would tell him anything, and his leadership style would prevent him from seeking advice.

4.6.2.2   Laissez-faire leadership style

The master remains completely passive and allows other crewmembers total freedom in their decisions. He makes only few suggestions. He neither makes negative nor positive judgments. The atmosphere is relaxed and communication concentrates on a variety of subjects, probably not all professional. In brief, this is a highly demagogic style of leadership whose prime aim is to please the other party, without necessarily concentrating on voyage objectives.

This situation frequently arises when the master is working with competent officers. The risk in this situation is a reversal of authority. One of the officers may be tempted to progressively take over, particularly because he or she would possibly like more autonomy and more initiative (considering himself or herself as a potential master).

4.6.2.3   Self-centered leadership style

The self-centered leadership style could characterize the whole bridge team: all work on their own, with their own plans, own focus of attention, and with very little communication about what they do. This situation is a dangerous threat to safety. It leads to misunderstandings and has a built-in lack of information sharing. The sharing of information is crucially important in an emergency situation, and absence of information sharing in this leadership style will often lead to problems.

4.6.2.4   Democratic leadership style

The democratic captain will consult his or her officers, asking them for their opinion prior to important decisions. The officers will perceive this as an encouragement to contribute and give their opinions. The authority gradient is flat and discussions are welcome. There is a high sharing of information. Democratic leadership style could turn into laissez-faire style, and it is therefore important that the captain is engaged in the discussions, making arguments, and demonstrating his or her own preferences and opinions clearly.

4.6.2.5   Leadership style summary

Which leadership style is the best? It depends on the situation. It is always important that the crew work together to create synergy. Synergy is obtained when the whole crew works together as a team, supporting each other through communication and the sharing of information. The democratic leadership style facilitates the creation of synergy and is therefore the preferred style under normal circumstances. But it can, under certain circumstances, be necessary to deviate from this democratic leadership style and move into, for example, the autocratic style (e.g., in the case of an emergency). A good leader possesses the ability to change leadership style according to the situation and thereby take advantage of the strengths of the most suitable leadership styles and avoid any negative side effects.

4.7   Conclusion

The objective of this chapter has been to illustrate some important concepts and models in relation to communication and teamwork. The focus was on the interaction between the individual and the group in a maritime socio-technical system. The issues covered in the first part of the chapter included characteristics of verbal communication, context and mutual understanding, closed-loop communication, social role and power, and some communication models. The second part of the chapter introduced two important concepts in relation to maritime teamwork: authority gradient and leadership style.

It is obvious that good communication and the appropriate leadership styles are essential for safety at sea. But this is not always easy to obtain. Communication can be disturbed in many ways; misunderstandings can occur, and roles and power could have negative influence on the efficiency of the communication. Leadership styles and authority gradient are heavily dependent on personalities—but also on cultural factors such as the so-called power distance, which is common in certain cultures and less significant in others. Culture is discussed further in Chapter 7.

chapter five

Work environment

5.1   Introduction

To state a truism, work, and all other human activities on a ship, always takes place within a physical environment. As described in the first chapter, the physical environment is one of the elements in the sociotechnical network that influences human performance. The focus of this chapter is on the interaction between the individual and the physical environment as illustrated in the sociotechnical system in Figure 5.1.

Many factors exist within a shipboard physical environment that can seriously compromise crew performance: these include factors such as noise,

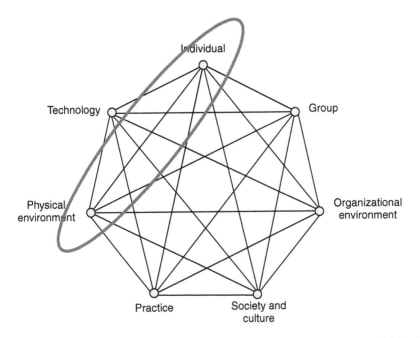

Figure 5.1 Interaction between individual and physical environment within the sociotechnical system model.

vibration, lighting, climatic conditions, and accommodation standards, as well as ship motions. Shortfalls within the physical environment such as excessive noise, living in confined spaces, and the sheer lack of privacy, all common to shipboard living, can exert a pervasive negative influence on crew. This negative impact may result in poor performance, physical and mental fatigue, or an increase in human error. In this chapter we focus on the following physical environmental aspects well known to influence the human element in the maritime domain:

1. Noise
2. Vibration
3. Lighting
4. Climatic conditions
5. Accommodation and social factors
6. Ship motion

It is crucial that all the above elements are given due consideration as early in the ship design process as possible. Each of these has an effect on operators' work performance (e.g., increased error rates), subjective comfort, safety (e.g., more accidents), and attitudes toward work and health (both long term and short term). In addition, the organization may also suffer losses, both through losing trained and qualified personnel and through workplace compensation costs.

5.2   Noise

5.2.1   Noise and sound

To give a definition, *noise* is often loosely described as "unwanted sound." *Sound* is really an auditory sensation that is due to pressure fluctuations of acoustic waves (oscillations about the ambient pressure of the atmosphere, consisting of longitudinal vibration of air molecules). For humans, it is a variation of pressure in the ear, which can be detected by receptor cells in the ear. The two most important characteristics for us are *frequency* and *intensity* (which correspond in lay terms to *pitch* and *loudness*). People vary in their interpretation of sound. Some people may label sound as noise, which might not be considered as noise by different people or in different situations.

In terms of frequency, humans are capable of detecting sound between 2 and 20,000 Hz (although at less than 16-Hz sounds are usually described as beats), but we are most sensitive to sound in the range of 2,000 to 5,000 Hz (roughly corresponding to the range of human speech). Sound intensity is often defined in terms of sound pressure level (SPL) and is measured in a logarithmic unit of decibels (dB). Because decibels are measured on a logarithmic scale, the relationship between decibels and sound intensity is not linear;

that is, 100 dB is not twice the intensity of 50 dB but 100,000 times the intensity, since a tenfold increase in intensity occurs with each 10-dB increase.

5.2.2 Noise exposure effects

In a shipboard environment noise can have varying effects, based on the sound level, frequency, and amplitude, as well as the task being performed. It is well known that unexpected intermittent noise is more disruptive than continuous noise, and high-pitched noise is often more distracting than low-pitched noise. At extreme levels, noise can be dangerous, causing partial or permanent deafness. At moderate intensities, noise is likely to affect performance. At low levels, noise can reduce comfort and increase annoyance (potentially influencing work performance through lowering of operator concentration and well-being).

A major source of noise on board ships comes from the main engines, propellers, maneuvering devices such as the steering gear, the auxiliary systems such as the heating ventilation and air conditioning (HVAC) units, cargo handling, and mooring equipment. Shipboard noise is also emitted through hull slamming.

The effects of noise can be described as both physiological and psychological. The most familiar physiological consequence is impairment of hearing. Other categories include:

- Increases in stress
- Decrements in performance
- Sleep disturbances
- Communication interferences

5.2.2.1 Hearing impairments

Noise-induced hearing impairment is considered one of the most prevalent irreversible occupational hazards. Excessive noise exposure gradually (or it can be quickly) damages the very small hair-like sensors deep in the inner ear. Noise is especially hazardous at the higher frequency range (between 3,000 and 6,000 Hz), with longer exposure times constituting a higher risk. Noise-induced hearing loss can be temporary (up to sixteen hours), called temporary threshold shift (TTS), or permanent, referred to as permanent threshold shift (PTS). In TTS, hearing returns to normal after a period of non-exposure to the noise that caused TTS. PTS can take years for its full effects to be entirely realized, but its effects are permanent. Factors that influence TTS and PTS include exposure duration (obviously, the longer the exposure, the higher the risk), exposure intensity (the louder the exposure, the higher the risk), and the type of noise (sometimes continuous noise can produce more TTS than does intermittent noise). As an example, damaging effects have been shown to occur above the 90 dB (A)* threshold. To avoid noise damage, it is sometimes recommended that for an eight-hour-per-day exposure, the equivalent noise level should not exceed 85 dB (A). Some classification societies have now set guidelines for safe exposure and noise level limits for shipboard operations (e.g., part of Germanischer Lloyd's (GL) Rules and Guidelines specify Required Noise and Vibration Limits for ships; these guidelines are publicly available on http://www.gl-group.com/infoServices/rules/pdfs/english/glrp-e.pdf).

5.2.2.2 *Increases in stress*

The psychological aspect of noise is more problematic to define due to its subjective nature. In general, however, noise acts as a stressor in the work environment and is annoying to most people. The stress factor may increase due to the problems that noise generates in communication and may take the form of frustration and anxiety over message comprehension and the need for repetitions.

5.2.2.3 *Decrements in performance*

Research studies that looked at the effects of noise on performance and safety showed that noise may produce some task impairment and increase error rates in the workplace. The severity of this problem depends on the type of noise (e.g., whether the noise is intermittent or continuous) and on the tasks being performed (e.g., whether simple or complex tasks). As shown in Chapter 2, it is evident that when a task involves auditory signals, for example, speech, noise levels of sufficient intensity that mask or interfere with the perception of these communication signals also interfere with performance of such tasks. This is especially true for sudden, unexpected noise, which causes distraction and may interfere with some tasks. In addition to the direct effects on performance, noise also has lasting aftereffects on cognitive performance with tasks such as reading, attention, problem solving, and memory most likely worsened.

5.2.2.4 *Sleep disturbances*

Research shows that high levels of noise pollution delay the onset of sleep, increase waking up during sleep periods, and generally interfere with rest, thus reducing the amount and quality of sleep. Furthermore, the louder the background noise, the more disturbing is its effect on sleep. On ships, crewmembers are constantly exposed to shipboard noise at all hours of the day. Sleep interruption due to noise is hence a common occurrence. Sleep

---

* ISO standards utilize a weighting sound level factor to use as a measure of loudness. Three weighted factors are currently in use referred to as dB (A), (B), and (C). These are usually expressed as curves with loudness (dB) plotted against frequency. They provide an indication of the sound energy filtered out in each frequency range. The curve of weighted sound level in dB (A) is the most commonly used.

interruption that brings about sleep debt (i.e., the cumulative effects of loss of sleep over several days) may lead to fatigue and performance problems. And as indicated in Chapter 3, studies of accidents often find operator fatigue somehow involved. Measures aimed at reducing sleep disturbance during the sleep period are crucial for reducing noise-induced sleep problems.

5.2.2.5   *Communication interferences*

Noise can certainly have a profound effect on verbal communication as highlighted in Chapter 2. Noise interferes with speech intelligibility and other communication tasks by adversely affecting the signal-to-noise ratio. Apart from speech, noise can also mask other signals such as alerts and warnings. For example, noise levels of 78 dB (A) can make conversations very difficult over a distance of one meter. As the sound pressure level of an interfering noise increases, people automatically raise their voice to overcome the masking effect upon speech (by increasing vocal effort). This can be both annoying and distracting and in most cases imposes an additional strain, which has been shown to lead to problems with concentration, fatigue, stress, decreased working capacity, misunderstandings, and problems in personal relations.

5.2.3   *Protection strategies*

Obviously, noise on a ship is almost ubiquitous. However, there are a variety of strategies that can be used to protect against high levels of noise, and much progress has been made over the years in reducing noise levels on merchant ships. From most effective (but generally more costly) to least effective (but often cheaper to implement) they are:

1. Reduce noise at source
2. Reduce noise exposure
3. Use noise management strategies

5.2.3.1   *Reduce noise at source*

One way to reduce noise at its source is to decrease the noise characteristics of a system. This is usually the most costly method but can also be the most effective. Installing equipment that is quieter and better built on board is costly but will in the long run result in reduced operating and maintenance costs. If this option proves too costly, an effective alternative to reduce noise at source includes such measures as protective planning (e.g., enclosing the source of the noise in a housing, using noise-absorbent insulation materials, and locating shipboard accommodation and living areas away from noisy machinery spaces).

5.2.3.2   *Reduce exposure*

When noise levels cannot be reduced at the source, or people cannot be isolated from the noise, proper use of personal protection (e.g., ear plugs/muffs) equipment should be implemented. Today's requirement for personal hearing protection, specifically for values in the 85-dB region (or lower), has made cases of severe unprotected exposures less common. Active noise-canceling systems are now being considered for limited areas where it is too difficult or costly to reduce the noise at the source. Other exposure reduction methods are to vary tasks that operators are undertaking, so that they are exposed to noise for a limited amount of time.

5.2.3.3 Management strategies

Noise exposure hazards have now been largely managed through continuous monitoring of onboard noise by the crew, through periodic medical examinations, through designing quieter ship machinery, reducing exposure, or requiring noise protection equipment to be used. Today, regulations for occupational noise exposure are almost globally enforced and the risk of exposure to occupational noise is thus minimized. Even so, many crewmembers who are exposed to general shipboard noise over a full career can expect to suffer some form of hearing loss in addition to the natural deterioration associated with aging.

5.3 Vibration

5.3.1 Whole body vibration

In reality we know that it is very difficult to avoid vibrations on board ships. Shipboard vibration is a result of excitation from machinery and propulsion systems, which can invariably lead to both high- and low-frequency perturbations. Apart from ship machinery, another source of particularly uncomfortable vibrations is hull slamming, which is produced as a result of the ship dropping from the top of a wave into a trough, and is influenced by the level of sea state (such as swell and wind-induced wave components) and ship speed (i.e., the higher the speed, the higher the slamming threshold speed). These lead to what is commonly referred to as whole body vibration, usually transmitted to the body through the buttocks, feet, and hands, which are the body parts most frequently in contact with vibrating surfaces.

Whole body vibration has been shown to affect comfort and performance, in some cases leading to additional chronic health problems such as back pain, musculoskeletal disorders (as already noted in Chapter 3), and temporary physiological changes. The effects may be immediate, occurring during a person's actual exposure, or they may be cumulative. For example, years of exposure to vibration have been shown to contribute to disorders or injuries of the lower back. In addition, vibration can cause fatigue and may contribute to increased error and accident rates. Vibration can also affect human performance indirectly. For example, if equipment in the visual field is vibrating, this may cause some blurring of vision with difficulties in reading and interpretation.

5.3.2   *Measuring vibration*

Similar to sound, vibration is usually expressed in terms of frequency and magnitude. Vibration occurs when a body moves in what is described as an oscillating motion about a reference position. The number of times a complete cycle takes place during a period of one second is called the *frequency* and is expressed in hertz. Research shows that human subjective sensitivity is more evident in the 4- to 8-Hz frequency range; nevertheless in one way or another, vibrations ranging from 1 to 20 Hz can affect human performance negatively. Frequencies below 1 Hz are further associated with such symptoms as motion sickness, covered later on in this chapter. Hence, frequency range usually determines the manner in which vibration affects comfort, performance, and health.

Vibration amplitude is commonly used to measure the magnitude of vibration severity. This can be quantified in several ways. Figure 5.2 shows two measures of amplitude, the *peak* and the *root-mean-square* (rms) amplitude. Peak amplitude is the largest positive or negative value in the acceleration time history relative to the mean. The rms acceleration (a calculated value) is the primary quantity used for expressing vibration magnitude as it accounts for the time history of the wave and also provides an amplitude value directly related to the energy content and, therefore, the destructive abilities of the vibration. This is measured in meters per second squared (m/s^2). At the most intense frequency range of 4 to 8 Hz, levels of 10 m/s^2 rms (for seated subjects) and 12 m/s^2 rms (for standing subjects) are considered very severe, while levels beyond 15 m/s^2 rms (for seated subjects) and 17 m/s^2 rms (for standing subjects) are considered as dangerous and intolerable (Kroemer and Grandjean 1997). It is, however, rare to encounter such acceleration levels on larger ships such as tankers and passenger ships; nonetheless such levels of acceleration have been known to occur on smaller vessels such as high-speed craft and small, fast boats.

Many attempts have been made to set safe and comfortable limits for human exposure to vibration based on research findings (Kroemer and Grandjean 1997). As indicated, these limits are usually expressed in terms of acceleration (rms) as a function of direction and frequency (Hz) as well as daily duration of exposure (usually expressed in hours and minutes).

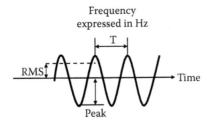

Figure 5.2   Measure of vibration in frequency and amplitude.

5.3.3   Protection strategies

Similar to noise, a number of protection strategies exist for reducing whole body vibration. Some protection strategies currently in use include:

- Limiting exposure time near or on a vibrating surface. In this regard, Kroemer and Grandjean (1997) provide the following guidelines when vibration becomes intolerable:
  - Below 2 Hz at accelerations of 30 to 40 m/s² rms
  - Between 4 and 14 Hz at accelerations of 12 to 32 m/s² rms
  - Above 14 Hz at accelerations of 50 to 90 m/s² rms
  These guidelines provide an indication of when vibration becomes intolerable, which means that from an ergonomic viewpoint the actual operating acceleration levels should be lower.
- Mechanically isolating vibrating sources or surfaces to reduce exposure
- Ensuring equipment is well maintained
- Installing vibration dampers

5.4   Lighting

5.4.1   Why we need to consider lighting

Similar to other environmental variables (such as noise and vibration) human factors consideration of lighting is vital. Symptoms of performing tasks under poor or inappropriate lighting include headaches, blurred/double vision, and lowering of visual performance. On board ships, illumination inadequacies may be present in confined or enclosed spaces, which may lead to visual performance problems when shipboard maintenance or routine work is required to be carried out. Adequate lighting is also crucial to ensure crew safety in emergency and evacuation situations.

5.4.2   Light, illumination, and luminance

Light is defined as electromagnetic energy. For humans, visible light is only a small part of the electromagnetic spectrum. The defining variables of light are similar to those of sound: intensity (corresponding to loudness/intensity with noise) and wavelength (corresponding to frequency/pitch with noise). Two important terms are employed in the study of light:

1. Illumination
2. Luminance

Illumination is the measure of the stream of light falling on a surface. This light may come from the sun, lamps, or other bright sources. It is measured in lux (lx). Illumination levels can vary from 2,000 to 100,000 lx in daylight and from 50 to 1,000 lx indoors.

Luminance is the measure of brightness of a surface; the perception of brightness of a surface is proportional to its luminance and the reflective power of the surface. Luminance is most frequently measured in units of candela per square meter (cd/m^2).

5.4.3   Indoor lighting

Light sources in most shipboard spaces usually comprise fluorescent tubes, with electric filament globes mainly restricted to accommodation and mess areas (used in combination with the fluorescent tubes). Filament lights are rich in red and yellow rays and emit heat. Fluorescent lighting is produced by passing electricity through a gas (e.g., argon or neon). The inside of the tube is covered with a fluorescent substance that converts the ultraviolet rays of the discharge into visible light. They have advantages over filament lights in terms of higher output and longer life, but have a problem with visible flicker (100 Hz).

The "best" (at least, most expensive) lamps try to imitate daylight incandescence to give a warm effect, as opposed to the harsh lighting obtained in some cheaper lamps. Studies with the more expensive lighting have produced mixed results, with these lamps preferred but with little work performance benefits. This brings us to the next topic of what is "good" lighting.

5.4.4   Visual comfort

What is a good visual environment for one person doing a specific job might be unsuitable for somebody else carrying out a different task. In general, for visual comfort and good optical performance the following requirements should be met.

5.4.4.1   Level of illumination

Fifty years ago illumination levels of 50 to 100 lx were recommended for workshops and offices; nowadays levels of 500 to 2,000 lx are recommended (Kroemer and Grandjean 1997). Higher levels of illumination are needed for tasks that are more visually demanding. An appropriate level of lighting (e.g., as specified under the U.S. DOD-HDBK-289 (SH) on lighting standards) is required where visual terminals are in use, such as the bridge.

5.4.4.2   Spatial balance of surface luminance

The even distribution of luminance over the environment is important for visual comfort and visibility. For example, on the bridge the provision of appropriate lighting becomes more complex as paper-based tasks, which may require higher levels of light, may need to be accomplished (e.g., chart work) together with monitoring visual displays, which may require lower levels of light than for the paper-based work. Generally, the larger the change of luminance across the environment, the greater the loss of visibility when moving between the different light levels. Task lighting should therefore be adjustable in light level and positioning, in order to reduce luminance disparity between paper-based documents and visual display terminals. In addition, lighting should allow positioning to avoid glare.

5.4.4.3   *Temporal uniformity of lighting*
Similarly, flicker can also be a potential problem with some lighting, especially fluorescent lights. Flicker is especially bad for younger workers and can cause problems such as headaches (and in extreme cases epileptic attacks). Providing "phase-shifted" lamps (e.g., two fluorescent lamps that flicker at slightly different times to create a more uniform light pattern) can help reduce the problem.

5.4.4.4   *Avoidance of glare with appropriate lights*
Inadequate lighting arrangements can be a further source of glare that makes viewing uncomfortable. Glare can be avoided by:

- reducing reflective surfaces (e.g., shiny floors)
- having no source of light in the visual field of the operator
- having lights fitted with shades/glare shields
- using fewer lamps of lower power
- angling the lights away both horizontally (over 30 degrees) and vertically (right angles) from the operator

5.4.4.5   *Summary*
In a human factors evaluation of the adequacy of the lighting environment on a ship we are interested in several factors:

- Is the lighting adequate for the tasks being undertaken?
- Is it spread evenly over the working area?
- Does it create glare and reflections that negatively influence performance?

Poor lighting, whether too bright or too dim, will have an adverse effect on performance and the physiological and psychological well-being of the operator. Although the human eye is able to adapt and function reasonably efficiently in a wide variety of lighting conditions, this adaptation causes strain and increases the potential for errors. The aim of good lighting, therefore, is to maximize performance while reducing eye strain on the operator.

5.5   Climatic conditions

As we just noted above, humans can adapt to a variety of environmental conditions; this also applies to variations in climate. However, on some occasions minor changes to our climatic environment can produce significant reactions that may have an impact on human performance and health. To some degree, we all intuitively know that the important components of climate include temperature and wind speed. More formally, the most important physical components of climate are:

1. Temperature
2. Humidity
3. Air movement
4. Air quality

We discuss each of these factors separately.

5.5.1   Temperature

The core temperature of the human body fluctuates a little around the 37 degrees Celsius (°C) mark (98.6 degrees Fahrenheit) (Kroemer and Grandjean 1997). When working indoors we rarely notice the air temperature if it is comfortable (on the bridge perhaps between 21 and 24 degrees Celsius (69.8–75.2 degrees Fahrenheit)). On most ships the indoor work environment is usually controlled to acceptable levels of temperature and humidity by the use of heating, ventilation, and air conditioning (HVAC) units. If these deviate from a comfortable level, it starts attracting attention. The range of comfort is fairly narrow, perhaps only 2 to 3 degrees Celsius (35.6–37.4 degrees Fahrenheit). However, big differences in comfort exist due to factors such as different operators' perceptions of a comfortable temperature, time of year, time of day, amount of physical work undertaken, and clothing worn. Hence, when designing ship ventilation systems, it is imperative to take into consideration the needs of personnel living and working aboard the ship as well as the work processes performed in particular spaces. With respect to temperature of surrounding surfaces, as a general rule, surfaces (e.g., a computer keyboard or a handheld tool) should not differ by more than ±3 degrees Celsius (±37.4 degrees Fahrenheit) from the air temperature.

5.5.2   Humidity

Humidity (the amount of moisture in the air) can vary in the range of 30 percent to 70 percent without causing thermal discomfort. Below 30 percent is too dry an atmosphere, which can cause ear, nose, and throat problems (e.g., irritation of the nasal passages). Over 70 percent rarely occurs in indoor work, although there may be exceptions to this in ship galleys and engine rooms.

5.5.3   Air movements

Air movements above 0.5 meters per second (m/s) are often experienced as unpleasant in an indoor work environment, such as the bridge. Especially unpleasant are air current from behind, currents on the neck and feet (especially sensitive), and cool draughts (even 2 to 3 degrees Celsius (35.6–37.4 degrees Fahrenheit) below the comfort zone) are more unpleasant than warm ones with airflows in excess of 0.2 m/s experienced as uncomfortable (Kroemer and Grandjean 1997).

5.5.4   Air quality

Odors, pollution, excessive water vapor, and excessive carbon dioxide can all cause discomfort. Commercial ships emit air pollutants under two major modes of operation: while underway and at berth (under auxiliary power). Emissions underway come from a ship's engine exhaust and are influenced by a great variety of factors including engine size, the fuel used (heavy fuel oil or diesel oil), operating speed, and load. Such pollutants can be harmful to crew even in low doses. As a general guide an operator on a ship requires about 30 cubic meters of fresh air per hour, more if tobacco is being smoked nearby or if physical work is being performed.

5.5.5   Body temperature regulation

As we have previously seen, the core temperature of a human adult needs to be maintained within a narrow range around the 37°C (98.6 degrees Fahrenheit) mark. Muscle contraction is the main source of heat within the body. The metabolism process (converting food into bodily mechanical energy) is a rather inefficient process, giving off substantial amounts of heat (80 percent heat, and 20 percent muscular energy).

The core body temperature is not constant; at night body heat drops by about 0.5°C (32.9°F), whereas intense sports (e.g., a marathon) can take the core temperature up to almost 40°C (104°F). Similarly, different parts of our body are usually at different temperatures; the skin is usually a few degrees cooler.

Although humans usually have good regulatory mechanisms, *hyperthermia* may occur if the body's core temperature rises above 41°C (105.8°F) (other effects include irritability, loss of concentration, loss of efficiency, increased errors/accidents, loss of performance in heavy work, and intense fatigue). *Hypothermia* may develop if body temperature falls below 35°C (95°F) (other less catastrophic effects of low temperatures include less mobility in the hands/feet, manual skills slowing down, increased clumsiness, and decreased touch sensitivity). Body temperature depends on several factors:

- Metabolism and the core temperature
- Regulatory control mechanisms: Blood flow, sweating, and shivering

- Climate: Air temperature, radiant temperature, humidity, and air movement
- Clothing
- Rate/type of work
- Individual differences (such as age and gender)

5.5.6 Management of heat and cold stress

Most of the time shipboard crewmembers are required to perform their duties indoors under climate-controlled conditions. However, it should be mentioned that many shipboard spaces contain environments of high heat and humidity, including machinery spaces, galleys, and laundries. Sometimes, shipboard work needs to be performed outdoors in either high or low temperatures (e.g., while mooring and unmooring or conducting boat drills in either a hot Australian summer or a cold Canadian winter), placing crew at increased risk of heat or cold stress. Hence, for tasks that must be performed outdoors, appropriate clothing should be worn and exposure to adverse climates both indoors and outdoors should be limited.

5.5.6.1 Heat stress

Heat stress occurs under high temperature environments. Effects of heat stress include increase in error rate with a general deterioration in performance due to a lack of movement precision. High relative humidity increases the risk of heat stress as it prevents sweat evaporation, the body's natural heat disposal mechanism. Heat stress can cause heat rash, fainting, heat cramps, heat exhaustion, and heat stroke. Heat stroke is very serious and can cause death, even in young and healthy individuals. Some of the techniques for the management of heat stress are summarized below (adapted from Kroemer and Grandjean 1997):

- Reduce relative humidity by using dehumidifiers (can be expensive)
- Increase air movement by fans or air conditioners
- Remove heavy clothing; permit loose-fitting, light-colored apparel
- Provide for lower energy expenditure levels (e.g., automate parts of the task or extend the time allowed to complete the task)
- Rotate personnel; schedule frequent rest pauses
- Schedule work to avoid extreme high temperature periods (e.g., avoid the midday sun)
- Select personnel who can tolerate extreme heat
- Permit gradual acclimatization to outdoor heat (approximately 2 weeks)
- Maintain hydration by drinking water and, if necessary, taking salt tablets
- Design for proper temperature control and utilize better technology to avoid or reduce heat stress conditions aboard ships

5.5.6.2   Cold stress

Extreme cold causes manual operations, particularly those requiring fine motor skill, to degrade. When the body is unable to warm itself, serious cold-related illnesses and injuries may occur, and permanent tissue damage and death may result. Some of the techniques for the management of cold stress are summarized below (adapted from Kroemer and Grandjean 1997):

- Provide portable heating units
- Increase body insulation by clothing appropriate to the temperature
- Require moderate energy expenditure; avoid rest that allows the body to cool down too much
- Avoid long exposure periods; rotate personnel
- Schedule work to avoid extreme cold temperature periods (e.g., avoid the middle of the night)
- Provide protection from wind at extreme temperatures
- Select personnel who can tolerate extreme cold
- Permit gradual acclimatization to outdoor cold
- Provide warm liquids for consumption

5.6   Accommodation and social factors

It is a fact of life that most human basic/primary needs are the same, regardless of the domain in which they work. People share basic needs for sleep, food, comfort, and social interaction. Some research in this area has shown that there is a clear link between shipboard comfort and contentment aboard ships (Hardwick 2000). Apart from affecting job performance, crew comfort or lack of it may influence the recruitment and retention of seagoing personnel. Hence, in addition to the operational requirements of the ship/organization, living spaces should reflect the personal and social needs of the crewmembers and provide them with an adequate level of off-duty facilities for individual privacy and social relaxation.

Living standards also need to consider the physical dimensions of the crew (anthropometry was discussed in Chapter 3). In today's global shipping organization this may be a problematic issue as crew can hail from a diversity of countries, making this dimensional aspect a bit more difficult to apply. The physical dimensions of crewmembers from developed countries have generally increased over the last century, due to such aspects as improved living conditions, medical care, and diet, with this trend expected to continue.

In general, primary social factors that need to be adequately considered on board ships include the following:

1. Sleeping accommodation, which needs to consider sleeping berth dimensions for maximum flexibility, comfort, and provide personal stowage requirements
2. Dining areas
3. Adequate privacy and relaxation facilities
4. Communication with family and friends back home (as discussed in Chapter 3)
5. High level of hygiene; toilets, bathrooms, and laundry facilities
6. Adequate facilities for recreation, fitness, and study.

5.7   Ship motions

During the early design stages of any vessel, an important aspect that should be taken into account is its sea-keeping characteristics (i.e., the way the vessel behaves under various environmental conditions). Good sea-keeping characteristics allow the vessel to perform most of its operational requirements successfully, even in the most adverse environmental conditions. It also minimizes ship motions. Ship motions can have an impact on such factors as crew effectiveness and safety and the ability to undertake specific tasks and activities. It is well known that ship motion results in feelings of seasickness, loss of motivation, decrements in performance, and fatigue, which can adversely affect accomplishment of tasks and overall operational requirements. Ship motion is associated with three primary consequences: (1) seasickness, (2) motion-induced interruptions, and (3) motion-induced fatigue. These effects are discussed next.

5.7.1   Seasickness

Seasickness is one of the most obvious and disconcerting effects of ship motion. It is also the most widely studied. Seasickness is known to occur when a person is not adapted to the motion response of the vessel. Studies have shown that the primary symptom of seasickness is nausea with signs consisting of general feelings of discomfort such as sweating, stomach awareness, pallor, and vomiting (Wertheim 1998). Other associated responses, reported to some degree, include apathy, headaches, increased salivation, and prostration.

One theory postulates that motion sickness comes about as a result of a conflict that arises between different body sensory systems, described in Chapter 2 (such as inner ear, visual, and vestibular senses), in a moving environment. So, for example, if the inner ear's signal to the brain does not match the visual or vestibular senses, seasickness is likely to occur. Hence, looking at the horizon while experiencing seasickness alleviates its effect to some extent, as it provides a visually stable cue for the brain to match up to the other sensory signals. There is also a psychological component associated with seasickness. Some people develop a sense of anxiety, sometimes even before boarding a ship, perhaps due to previous experience with motion stimuli. This may eventually develop into feelings of discomfort or nausea when exposed to certain provocative motions. Studies indicate that feelings of seasickness usually occur at low frequency pitch and roll motions below the 0.3 Hz range in combination with vertical acceleration magnitudes between 1 and 4 m/s² rms.

Sensitivity to seasickness varies widely among humans, in that a number of people may be more prone to seasickness than others. Lawther and Griffin (1988) collected data on seasickness using a questionnaire survey from over 20,000 passengers traveling on six passenger ships, two hydrocrafts, and a hydrofoil together with 370 hours of ship motion recordings. Their combined results showed that 7 percent of passengers vomited at some time during the voyage, with 21.3 percent indicating that they felt *slightly unwell*, 4.3 percent stating that they felt *quite ill*, and 4.1 percent indicating that they felt *absolutely dreadful*. Generally, research has shown that up to 30 percent of people may suffer some form of seasickness during normal sea conditions, with this figure rising dramatically in rough seas (to around 50 to 90 percent). On merchant ships this may represent a significant loss in personnel, which may be more of an issue today due to reduced crewing. Providing a more positive outlook, people commonly adapt to ship motions following long exposure, which may provide some relief from the original discomfort. However, this is not always the case with some people never really recovering from seasickness while in a moving environment.

5.7.2   Motion-induced interruptions

Motion-induced interruption (MII) occurs when the vessel's motion causes a loss of balance in the person's stance thereby interrupting task(s) being performed. This is associated with attempting to maintain stability to try and minimize work disruptions. MII is predicted based on a model that records the number of times loss of balance occurs while standing in a moving environment. Results are expressed as the number of MIIs per minute. Some research in this area focuses on predicting MII safe limit criteria for a shipboard environment. Some classification societies (such as Lloyd's Register and Det Norske Veritas) specify MII safe limit criteria for some shipboard spaces that should not be exceeded.

5.7.3   Motion-induced fatigue

Ship motion is also associated with motion-induced fatigue (MIF), which is related to energy expenditure to preserve balance and to walk around in a moving environment. The extra effort that is exerted to retain balance may accelerate feelings of physical fatigue. Overall, MIF is likely to have a large impact on many aspects of performance. Research in MIF is not that widespread at the moment, as work in this area has tended to focus more on MII.

The AABCD (Australian, American, British, Canadian, and Dutch) working group on Human Performance at Sea has done some research work in the area of MIF, and its agenda dictates that it will continue to do so. Another aspect worth mentioning is the indirect effect of ship motion, which is associated with sleeping problems, as mentioned earlier in this chapter.

5.7.4   Prevention strategies

To manage and reduce risks associated with negative effects of ship motions on performance it is important that potential solutions are developed and tested. Prevention strategies can basically be divided into two approaches. The first approach is to alter the design characteristics of the vessel to minimize exposure to uncomfortable frequency and acceleration levels that lead to motion-induced problems. This involves, for example, consideration of location of key workspaces and living areas during the early design stage. Hence, with further additional effort at the design stage, the comfort of the crew can be greatly improved, for example, by locating crew work and some living spaces in areas of lower acceleration. In addition, exploration at an early design stage of hull forms that, in association with the predicted sea and ship motions, is particularly important in avoiding this problem. This is the most desirable approach, which can immensely improve the comfort of the crew. However, there is a limit to how much it can alleviate seasickness effects. It is also important to note that most mariners are working on older vessels, designed with no consideration of motion-related issues, which bring us to the second approach.

The second approach is to utilize a management approach. One way may involve the use of seasickness medication. This approach, however, introduces a number of problems: some seasickness medications lead to undesirable side effects in addition to some form of desensitization, which may be a health hazard particularly if crewmembers are operating potentially hazardous equipment. Other management approaches used to ease the effects of seasickness include serving nongreasy, fresh healthy foods, focusing on the horizon while at sea (as previously mentioned), and lying down if discomfort or nausea is experienced. Another approach is to allow time for habituation by going out to sea initially in low sea state conditions whenever possible. This will provide time for the crew to adapt to ship motion stimuli.

5.8   Physical environment standards

A number of standards currently exist that cover some aspects of the shipboard physical environment. These, however, mainly deal with ensuring that a level of health and safety is maintained and refrain from providing necessary data aimed at maintaining a level of performance and comfort. Current maritime standards available in this area can be split into international and national standards.

Noise and vibration standards can be considered one of the first developments in this area. To minimize short- and long-term health effects, requirements and guidance on noise and vibration standards provide allowable
limits for most working and living spaces aboard ship. These have been
incorporated into various maritime standards by the major classification
societies, the International Maritime Organization (IMO) and the International Standard Organization (ISO). For example, IMO resolution A468 (XII):
1981 (Code on Noise Levels on Board Ships) and ISO 2923: 1996-12 (Acoustics—Measurements of Noise on Board Vessels) essentially deal with recommendations concerning noise measurements and limits aboard ship. Some
of the major classification societies and ISO 6954: 2000E (Mechanical Vibration—Guidelines for the Measurement, Reporting and Evaluation of Vibration with Regard to Habitability on Passenger and Merchant Ships) deal with
vibration limit values for a shipboard environment.

As indicated earlier, consideration of appropriate lighting for specific tasks
and/or activities is very important. Lighting requirements on board ships,
whether conducting maintenance, visual tasks (such as tracking and looking
at VDT), or simply reading, do not vary much from the requirements of similar shore-based tasks or activities. In this regard, most lighting standards can
be found in general human factors sources. Some maritime-specific lighting standards are available, such as the U.S. Navy Shipboard Habitability
Design Criteria. Shipboard emergency lighting is covered under IMO Resolution A.752 (18) and also within the International Convention for the Safety
of Life at Sea (SOLAS). An important aspect to consider when selecting the
most appropriate lighting standards is to ensure that these match similar
shipboard tasks. Examples of lighting standards can be found in the U.S.
DOD-HDBK-289 (SH) Military Handbook: Lighting on Naval Ships (Metric)
and the U.S. Navy Shipboard Habitability Design Criteria as already mentioned above.

Crew accommodation standards are mainly found under the International
Labour Organization (ILO) standards (e.g., ILO 92: 1949 (Revised) Accommodation of Crews Convention; ILO 147: 1978 Minimum Standards in Merchant
Ships Convention; ILO 68: 1946 Food and Catering (Ships' Crews) Convention (Article 5); and ILO 133: 1970 Crew Accommodation on Board Ship Convention (supplementary provisions)). Some of these standards such as ILO 92
have incorporated guidelines on adequate indoor climate characteristics such
as temperature, humidity, and air velocity in a marine environment. There
are also some national standards that account for crew accommodation and
these usually form part of flag state administration requirements (e.g., the
U.K. Merchant Shipping (Crew Accommodation) Regulations 1997).

With regard to ship motion, some of the major classification societies have
defined sea-keeping characteristics and performance standards for ships.
Two of the human factors criteria used for measuring the maximum allowable sea-keeping performance limits have been defined as (1) motion sickness incidence (MSI), which is measured as a percentage of personnel who

will vomit as a result of a given level and nature of ship motions, and (2) MII, which is measured as the incidence of personnel losing balance as a result of ship motions. It should be noted that MII calculations are currently based on the sliding or toppling of rigid bodies, rather than actual humans.

Despite the above maritime standards, to date the maritime industry lacks comprehensive guidelines on physical environment or habitability standards for ships. With a general global trend of crew reductions, the maritime domain has come to realize that new ways are required to attract and retain qualified seafarers. More emphasis on the shipboard physical environment seems to be a useful attraction for the recruitment and retention issues currently plaguing this industry. A recent publication by one of the major classification societies, the American Bureau of Shipping (ABS), is a welcome addition to the much-needed consolidated guidelines on crew habitability for ships (Guide for Crew Habitability on Ships, 102-HAB). This guide incorporates most aspects dealing with crew physical environment (noise, vibration, lighting, climate, and accommodation) into one document, and is a big step in the right direction.

5.9 Conclusion

In this chapter, the effects of some aspects of the physical environment on task performance and crew health have been presented. When the physical environment in which shipboard crew live and work exceeds known and established limits it can directly affect crew performance, health, and well-being.

It should be evident that protecting crew health, comfort, and well-being by paying more attention to the physical environment also results in improved task performance, a reduction in errors and accidents, and potentially greater retention of experienced crew.

chapter six

Interacting with technology

6.1 Introduction

This chapter begins by giving a brief overview of why it is important to consider technology/individual interaction factors, and then it introduces some human-related issues in the design, standardization, and integration of maritime equipment. Following that, it considers human responses to technology, before reviewing in more detail the issue of operator situation awareness and technology. Finally, it makes some concluding remarks and comments on further work required in this area.

As illustrated in Figure 6.1, the focus of this chapter is on the interaction between individual and technology within the sociotechnical system model.

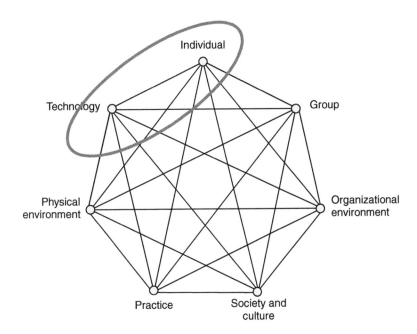

Figure 6.1 The sociotechnical system model focusing on technology/individual interaction factors.

6.2   Importance of human–machine interaction in maritime safety

The technology/individual interaction factor is one of the principal parts of the sociotechnical model described in Chapter 1. This is because most of the work carried out on a ship involves operators interacting with some kind of technology. Often the technology is quite simple (such as paper and pen, or a spanner); however, since the 1960s the technology has become increasingly complex. This change accelerated in the early 1990s with the increasing use of computers, communication, and navigation equipment such as Global Positioning Systems. The trend seems likely to continue, and automation on ships will undoubtedly become even more widespread. Optimizing this technology so that it matches the individual operator's skills, capabilities, and limitations, and integrating the technology within the system of work aboard a ship are therefore key issues to consider. With that in mind, we begin by considering some problems, opportunities, and challenges on ships with human–machine interaction (HMI).

6.3   Types of HMI problems on ships

There can be many HMI issues on board ships. The seriousness of the issues range from aspects that might cause very minor inconveniences (e.g., an infrequently used control for some non-safety-critical element located in a slightly inappropriate place) to issues that in certain circumstances may cause either serious problems with the safety or efficiency of the whole ship or may result in injuries and accidents to the individual operator. Some examples of these HMI problems (which have varying degrees of seriousness depending on the exact situation) are:

- Lack of equipment standardization
- Lack of equipment usability (including information overload issues)
- A new device that is essentially irrelevant to the task
- Poor ergonomic design of equipment
- Inadequate operator training and support
- Over-reliance on the technology by operators
- Rapid change in technology without it being fully integrated
- Ignoring human factors aspects in the design and deployment of the technologies
- Deterioration of skills of the individual operators from the introduction of new equipment

Maritime equipment of many generations is often together on the bridge, as illustrated in Figure 6.2, old VHF radio and modern radar equipment. New equipment is often added to an old bridge wherever it may fit.

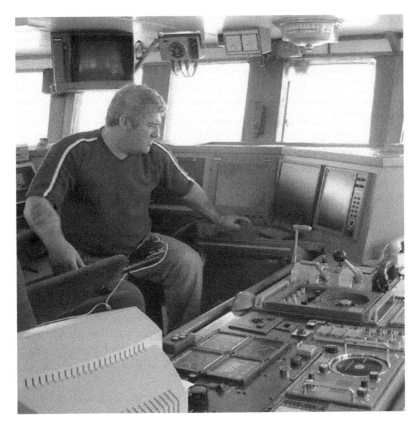

Figure 6.2   Many generations of maritime equipment on the bridge.

Many of these issues were present when the passenger ship *Royal Majesty* grounded in 1995 after the Global Positioning System antenna cable became partly disconnected. This resulted in erroneous information being displayed on the automated system, with none of the crew noticing. Among the factors purportedly involved were inadequate training standards when using an integrated bridge system (IBS), inadequate standards for design, testing, and installation of the IBS, and too much trust/over-reliance in the technology (so ignoring or not using other sources of information). Many of these issues are covered in this chapter. We set the scene by considering three overarching areas in more depth below.

6.3.1   Lack of equipment standardization

To move away from the maritime environment for one moment, a simple example of the lack of standardization is which side of the road cars use for driving; a large number of countries use the left side (e.g., the United Kingdom, Australia, India, and Japan) and another large number use the right side (e.g., France, the United States, Germany, and Canada). Of course, although it is theoretically possible to change the side used (as happened in Sweden in the twentieth century), it is unlikely to happen today. The side of road used for driving also has knock on effects for the design of the vehicle: equipment: most obviously this dictates which side the steering wheel is located on, but more indirectly it influences placement of other equipment such as indicators, light switches, and the fuel tank.

Returning to the maritime environment, human factors data are of limited worth if they are not applied to the design, deployment, or evaluation of jobs, systems, products, or tasks. One method of applying such data is in the form of standards, regulations, and guidelines. Many standards and guidelines are applicable to maritime operations and to the equipment used on board ships, for example, the American Bureau of Shipping guidance on bridge and navigation equipment design. Similarly, the IMO regularly produces guidelines of key human factors issues; two examples of recent topics include guidance for the use of IBS (e.g., Maritime Safety Committee Circular 1061 (2003) covering aspects such as operator training, emergency procedures, and testing systems before full operational use) and issues to consider when introducing new technologies on ships (e.g., Maritime Safety Committee Circular 1091 (2003) covering aspects such as standardization and considering how automation changes the task and the operator's performance). Clearly, these are important topics, which are largely covered in this chapter.

Most standards applicable to maritime operations deal with fairly simple environmental, equipment, and task stressors (such as noise levels over a working day) rather than complex cognitive activities involving new technologies on ships. The number of standards and regulations that specifically exist for maritime automation is low: the main regulations come from the IMO, such as the SOLAS Chapter 5, Regulation 15 (which covers features such as bridge design and navigational systems). The IMO guidelines to support this regulation cover key issues such as bridge layout, environment, workstation layout, alarms, displays, and controls. Similarly, the IMO has produced reasonably easy to follow submission templates for owners to show that major refits or new builds support the aims of the regulation.

It is not the place here to review all possible standards concerning maritime equipment and operations, but often bridge operators are faced with equipment originally from several different suppliers—where each supplier uses its own standards, causing the total bridge system to lack consistency. Likewise, navigation and engine equipment can vary greatly between ships, so operators may need to adjust regularly to different layouts; such variation is a fertile source of error (especially when accompanied by reduced crewing levels). For example, U.S. National Transport Safety figures (quoted by Rowley et al. 2006) found that nearly one third of maritime accidents were due to poor design of equipment (for which lack of standardization is a factor).

However, in theory, having international (e.g., ISO or IMO) rather than purely national standards (e.g., American, British, or Japanese) allows multinational manufacturers to make one maritime product that will be sold all over the world (e.g., Portable Pilot Units, which can reduce the need for a pilot to become familiar with a ship's navigational and other equipment when entering a port). Given the international aspect of maritime operations today, this can produce large cost savings, and often has usability benefits for the maritime consumer.

The overall picture is, however, complicated. In addition to the existence of well-formulated and legally enforceable standards and regulations, other "human factors good practices" also exist (such as Human Factors Integration plans). Additionally, some standards exist for only limited maritime occupations. A good example of this is Military Standards, which are usually only applicable in the military context. The U.S. Department of Defense and the U.K. Ministry of Defence have both produced highly detailed documents that cover a plethora of human factors design guidelines and approaches. These cover issues such as user-centered design, workspace design, lighting, controls, and designing for maintainability. Although such military standards and guidelines are undoubtedly worthy, they are often substantial documents of many hundred pages with requirements that could be expensive to implement, and are probably often not needed on commercial shipping. Thus, they might not be overly applicable to nonmilitary maritime companies or their equipment manufacturers. Therefore, it is hoped that this book will at least provide an overview of the types of human factors material they describe.

Most standards bodies rely on unpaid assistance by the various committee members; thus it can take a long time for standards to appear (up to ten years is not uncommon). For fast-moving industries like maritime navigation equipment design, standards are often well behind the technology, causing the standards to be very ineffective. Similarly, standards can be criticized for being too general (thus not precise enough for designers) or only establishing minimum requirements (often due to them being a compromise by the various committee members). Finally, existing equipment is often not standardized on ships in the same fleet, so full standardization may require retrofitting, a process that can be problematic and costly, so a longer-term goal of achieving appropriate standardization at the outset is usually preferable. For example, Electronic Chart Display and Information Systems (ECDIS) usually superimpose electronic charts, ship position, and radar onto one display. Although in theory such devices can improve navigation precision and reduce operators' mental workload, there is still a considerable variation between different ECDIS interfaces on different ships, so retraining and practice is required for operators needing to change between different devices.

However, when successful, standards can be exceedingly useful. In addition to the safety and efficiency benefits, standardization can also fit well into the process of conducting human factors audits. Audits can be used for purposes such as to assess the cost–benefit of different interventions, current safety practices, or future training requirements. The application of standards can also assist in maritime certification, compliance testing, and when developing and applying safety management systems. As we will see throughout this chapter, appropriate standardization of technologies can be a key human factors issue.

6.3.2   Lack of equipment usability

An issue related to standardization is equipment usability. Even if an article of maritime equipment is standardized, it does not necessarily mean that it is usable (or vice versa). Put very simply, usability means that the operators who use the product can do so quickly and easily to accomplish the required maritime tasks. Everything to do with a product has to be usable for operators who deal with it. This does not just refer to sophisticated new technologies, but also their documentation and maintenance. Similarly, usability applies equally to simple products such as hand tools. In many ways the benefits of usability are obvious, but can include increased maritime efficiency, fewer work injuries, improved operator acceptance, fewer errors, earlier detection of the requirement for maintenance, less required training, and fewer mistakes and violations. Maritime technology should not be seen as a "barrier," whereby the operator has to focus on the technology and not the task. Likewise, as much as possible, the technology should fit to the operator and the task, and not require the operator to fit the technology, but all too often operators need to adapt simply to get a job done.

The application of human-centered design principles can help to ensure the end product is usable. This essentially involves identifying who the operator is, what the product will be used for and how will the operator use it, what other systems/products are in place, how the product will integrate with the existing products, and how its successful design and deployment will be evaluated. Sadly, the usability testing of a technology is often undertaken only by a technology developer rather than the maritime organization or ship crew and management (shore or ship based) or a human factors practitioner. Assessing the needs for new equipment, seeing how it would be integrated with other work systems, and evaluating its successful introduction should all be undertaken where possible by involving the likely end users of the device.

6.3.3   Automation issues

New automation in the maritime domain is developed and deployed for a number of reasons, among which are the requirements for enhanced precision, fuel cost savings, more data/information, and reduced crewing. Much of the automation is being introduced onto the bridge, especially for ship navigation and related functions. Among the technologies being introduced are electronic navigation charts (ENC), electronic chart display and information systems (ECDIS), IBS, integrated navigation systems (INS), and automatic identification systems (AIS, for traffic management and to help avoid collisions). Likewise, such systems as operator fatigue detection technologies are being tested. Clearly, there is the potential for such systems to overload, confuse, and distract, rather than assist, an operator. Therefore, approaches like standardization, appropriate training, alarm integration, operator and manager consultation (both ship and shore based), input and feedback, and coordination by maritime authorities are all vital. Equally, using human factors principles to design the equipment, procedures, training, evaluation, and implementation of such systems is also of key importance.

To put the issue into context, we need to go back a few years. In the early 1950s, formal work regarding "allocation of function" between humans and machines was initiated. The impetus for this work was the growing complexity of systems, and the increasing use of automation, especially in aviation. Such automation often had negative consequences, for example, some aircraft in World War II that were unable to be flown safely due to poor ergonomics.

Essentially, the allocation of function approach made lists of tasks that machines/computers were good at (e.g., ability to perform repetitive, routine tasks) and tasks that people are good at (e.g., judgment, inductive reasoning). Thereafter, functions/tasks of a system were divided up based on who (person or machine) was the most appropriate to undertake them. Although the method had its critics (e.g., how is effective person/machine integration achieved), it has been widely used in both the process control and aviation domains. To some degree this trend is still in evidence today in the design principles to help maintain operator situation awareness (described in Chapter 2) in automated systems, in which recommendations are made concerning using automation to carry out routine actions and using humans for higher-order cognitive tasks (Endsley, Bolte, and Jones 2003).

A classic paper about some of the problems encountered with increased automation in the process control and aviation industries is that of Bainbridge (1983/87) who pointed out a series of "ironies of automation." These ironies show how automation of processes can often expand, rather than eliminate, problems with the human operator. They are also relevant to maritime operations. The types of ironies that Bainbridge lists include manual control skills (longer-term loss of skill of experienced operators, so when they need to intervene they are not as efficient), being "out of the control loop" (by the operator only passively monitoring an automated system, so when intervention is necessary the operator does not know the exact system state, which is often exacerbated by vigilance problems during monitoring), and negative operator attitudes to newly developed automation (often mistrust, resentment, and resistance to change). The core of the matter, according to Bainbridge, is that designers of systems often try to eliminate the human as much as possible, but still leave the operator to do the tasks that designers cannot work out how to eliminate.

Increasing pressures brought about by reduced crew numbers and the influence of increased automation have dramatically changed the role of the maritime operator. Automation can change the task it was meant to support, it can create new ways for human errors to manifest themselves (often because the effects of the errors are less directly visible, and the consequence of the error might not be immediate), and it can provide fewer opportunities for error detection and recovery. For example, deck officers are now expected to spend long periods on the bridge alone or with just a helm, with little to do other than monitor an increasing number of automated systems both on the bridge and some in the engine room, resulting in the removal of the human operator from the control loop of a particular system. Deck officers must be aware of the various functions of the different modes of the ARPA (Automated Radar Plotting Aid) display and how each mode is set up to navigate the ship safely, as well as keep track of which mode is active. In these conditions, the safety of the ship and its crew depends on the ability of the deck officer to maintain appropriate levels of alertness and vigilance. This can be very difficult, considering that the supervisory control task is specifically ill-suited to the cognitive capabilities of humans.

Therefore, although new automated systems can offer opportunities to reduce crew size, the work of Bainbridge and others suggests that introducing automation to replace operator weaknesses often compromises system safety rather than enhancing it.

6.4   Specific issues in the design and integration of maritime equipment

The above has given an overview of three generic maritime HMI problems. In the following section we examine some specific human factors issues with the design and integration of maritime equipment.

Chapter 2 of this book was concerned with perceptual factors. This is very relevant to the optimal design, deployment, and usage of maritime technologies, such as control panels (e.g., on bridges), engine monitoring systems, and general ship alarm signals. For example, perceptual factors are relevant not only in relation to the detectability of an alarm, but also because they can influence operators' cognitions (e.g., decisions) and actions (e.g., behavioral responses) in a variety of ways, often quite subtly.

Ship interface design should draw heavily on knowledge from both physical and cognitive ergonomics. Generally new maritime technologies require new ways of working, so care must be taken with many key human factors issues when introducing new devices and systems. Here we focus largely on advanced maritime technologies that are used on the bridge. First, we briefly review ship controls and displays, then we look at maritime warnings and alarms, and finally we examine in more depth an area of increasing current interest: E-Navigation.

6.4.1   Controls and displays

As anybody with even the briefest contact with the maritime industry knows, a wide range of different controls and displays exists on board a ship. These vary from computer keyboards and touch screens, to more traditional devices that have a more direct physical link between the action (control) and the shown consequence (displays), for example, turning a handle to open an equipment storage cupboard or a valve. Most controls are operated by an operator's hands, but a few manual interaction devices are foot controlled, especially those requiring larger forces, or when operators' hands are otherwise engaged. As well as the wide ranges of controls and displays on a ship, there is often a wide variation in the controls and displays used between ships, especially in the engine, bridge, and cargo areas (despite some standards existing).

Let us consider some first principles. How long it takes, and how difficult it is, for a crewmember to control an event on the ship is influenced by several factors: How complex is the decision to be made (more alternatives usually slow down the response), what the crewmember expects to happen (humans perceive and respond more rapidly and more accurately to expected information), how "compatible" the event is (the more compatible the event is with the required control response, the faster and more accurate it will be, e.g., when turning a car steering wheel to the right, the expectation is that the car will turn right), and whether any kind of feedback is given.

Another factor is familiarity with the ship's controls and displays. For example, the collision between the ferry *Pride of Portsmouth* and the frigate *HMS St. Albans* in 2002 was partly because crewmembers on the *Pride of Portsmouth* were unfamiliar with the controls (Rowley et al. 2006). Similarly, the U.K. container ship *Berit* grounded in the Baltic Sea in 2006 because crewmembers were not familiar with, and therefore did not use, the full functionality of the electronic charting system fitted.

People are visually dominant. Most of the information received and used by operators comes from their visual system. However, as indicated in Chapter 2, other senses also have a major part to play; for example, hearing for auditory warnings or smell for onboard fires. A frequently used distinction for displays is between dynamic and static information. Dynamic information on ships can include wind speed, stop/go lights, and engine pressure monitors. Computer text/graphics have traditionally been thought of as static information; however, the increasing use of display screens to show ship data parameters is blurring this distinction. Whatever the name, the relative advantages of different display types is a huge topic: for example, in displays showing numbered values, digital displays are often faster with more accurate readings, but less effective at helping an operator to detect direction/rate of change than their analogue counterparts. Much of the work on printed information displayed on computer screens examined such factors as font design, on screen text size, case (lowercase is usually easier to read), word order, and color (white on black or other color combinations). There is not the space here to review all these findings, but we will touch on several key aspects in the next section on warnings.

The compatibility of controls and displays (or stimulus and responses, in the language of experimental psychologists) is a major issue. Compatible controls and displays require fewer mental transformations, so take less time to respond to. There are two elements:

1. The location of the controls with respect to their corresponding displays.
2. The exact control responses that should be made in response to the displays.

The second element depends on the set of expectations that an operator has about how the display will respond to a control action. Ideally it should match the internal model the operator has, and also have movement compatibility. As a very simple example of movement compatibility, on small boats turning the tiller to the left should also move the rudder to the left.

Such discussion brings us to the subject of population stereotypes. Population stereotypes are developed largely from experience of natural phenomena or of cultural conventions. An example is reading direction: the Western stereotype is from left to right, but the Chinese stereotype is different. Population stereotypes can be useful in maritime design by placing constraints to how a device's controls and displays are designed: for example, it is sometimes recommended that scale numbers should increase from left to right, or clockwise. Likewise, stereotypes are less vulnerable to stress, so are useful in ship emergency operation. However, due to the international nature of ship operations (and the different crew nationalities) not everyone on board may share the same stereotype when interacting with a particular device.

To sum up, a large number of factors influence the effectiveness of ship controls and displays, and no single arrangement will be optimal for all situations. Only by considering the types of human factors data presented above, and through careful testing (involving end users), can the most advantageous designs be implemented. As a final point to make here, with the increasing trend toward one-man bridge operation and the increasing integration of the various shipboard navigation and piloting components, it is perhaps even more essential than ever that controls and displays are optimized.

6.4.2 Warnings and alarms

Warnings and alarms are essentially just a different kind of display. But given their importance to maritime operations they are treated as a special case here.

6.4.2.1 *Visual warnings*

Visual warnings are becoming more prevalent in many areas, due to more hazard awareness, greater safety concerns, and product liability issues; the maritime environment is no exception here. It is better to either design out a hazard or to provide protection against the danger. If this cannot be done, then to be effective, written warnings must be seen, read, understood, and heeded. As with other maritime artifacts, designing an effective warning involves iterative design and testing with the relevant operator population. Other factors that influence the effectiveness of warnings include crew motivation, compliance cost, and the abilities/skills of the individual operators. It should also be noted that warnings are often not very effective; often only a 10 percent compliance is obtained, and this can be less if the compliance cost is high, there are social pressures not to comply, or if they are presented at the wrong time or place.

It should be noted that maritime warning information does not just have to be text, as pictures, drawings, and symbols can also be used. Their relative advantages are:

- Often pictorial information is good for speed, but text is better for accuracy.
- Symbols can be of numerous types, and can have the advantages over text in that their legibility is better, they can be used for crewmembers who are either illiterate or not schooled in the primary written language on board the ship, and they generally produce faster reactions. But their success depends on the concept to be displayed; some things are quite difficult to display symbolically, for example, a symbol to warn of a hatch door being sometimes open.
- Generally the symbols that require much learning/training are less effective.

When symbols are used in the same context, standardization is essential, especially for symbols that require some learning. Some coding dimensions (to identify symbols within a certain class) include color, shape, and size. For example, with color coding it is usually possible for an operator to be able to distinguish up to nine different color types, but using fewer is preferable.

6.4.2.2 *Audible warnings (alarms)*

There are two main objectives that audible warnings must accomplish. First, they must attract attention; that is, they must be noticed (seen or heard) and they must be attended to. As indicated above for visual alarms, their position (e.g., central in the regular field of view), size, and intensity are very important. Flashing lights are typically better detected than static lights (but the rate of flashing should be within the limits of temporal sensitivity, and often flashing lights can cause annoyance if used for a noncritical warning). Likewise, for auditory alarms, loudness (intensity), pitch (frequency), and duration are all important, as is the alarm sounding at the correct time and place.

A critical factor is that warnings must provide understandable information needed for crew to make informed decisions that produce the correct response. There are many examples where shortfalls in onboard alarm systems led to accidents. One such example is the *Aquitaine* passenger ferry accident. In essence, the ferry collided with the berth due to a fault in the controllable pitch propeller (CPP). One of the contributory factors leading to this accident was shortfalls in the provision of an adequate warning system, which resulted in the engineers' inability to detect the fault in the shaft-driven pump of the faulty port CPP system. Had there been adequate warnings designed within the system, the engineers may have been alerted to the fact and corrective action taken in time. This accident is mentioned again in Chapter 7.

The IMO has produced some general guidance concerning type, function, and number of alarms required on board vessels. These documents, however, do not provide sufficient information to ensure that an integrated understanding of onboard alarm systems is made. The main problem is that too little research has gone into warning and alarm system design regarding how best to communicate and convey important information to the ship's crew. On board ships there are a large number of unique alarm systems, which can overwhelm the operator. For example, in ship bridges (or engine rooms) it is not uncommon to have forty different auditory and visual alarms. Apart from the large number of alarms, often these can be too loud and sound too frequently. In emergency/abnormal situations, it is possible that many of these alarms might sound at the same time, and too many alarms can reduce response performance by overloading the operator. Under such conditions, crewmembers may adopt an inappropriate alarm sampling strategy, or they may just ignore them.

No magic solutions are given here, but one approach is to match the saliency (in terms of the attention it is likely to attract) of an alarm with its level of criticality for the system. For example, alarms that are vital to the safe operation of a system are bigger and brighter (or louder) than those for less critical operations. So, testing individual device alarms in comparison to others and as part of the overall ship alarm system is vital.

6.4.3   E-Navigation

In this chapter we have already mentioned some new developments in maritime technologies and systems such as IBS. Here we introduce another emerging maritime topic, E-Navigation. E-Navigation (sometimes known as Enhanced Marine Navigation or simply E-Nav) can be defined as the coordinated collection, processing, integration, and display of maritime information, either aboard or ashore, by electronic means to enhance navigation, safety, and security, as well as protection of the environment. Successful

E-Nav will require comprehensive electronic navigation charts, fail-safe positioning signals, reliable transmissions (ship-to-ship, ship-to-shore, and shore-to-ship), optimized displays, and agreed ways to prioritize information (e.g., in an emergency situation). As such, it would use both existing and new navigation tools to develop a global system that would be useful for all ships. Of course, many previously mentioned existing navigational and communication technologies and services would be involved.

The possible benefits of E-Nav could be increased maritime safety, efficiency, security, and reliability; more standardized navigation procedures and training; cost savings; improved communication; fewer errors/incidents; access to relevant real-time information; environmental benefits (due to more efficient navigation and fewer accidents); and possibly even a more coordinated improvement of the dominant maritime culture (e.g., improving aspects of safety culture) through the widespread introduction of E-Nav. Thus, although no formal cost–benefit analyses are yet possible, the IMO believes that a coordinated action would result in the largest advantages, as opposed to individual actions undertaken piecemeal by local agencies (e.g., ports or coastal regulators).

However, such speculation is perhaps getting a little beyond the current reality. The exact scope of E-Nav, as well as the precise tools, policies, and overall standards required, has been widely discussed by the IMO and local agencies since 2005, but at the time of writing E-Nav is more of an interesting concept than a concrete approach. As yet, no broad, coordinated international strategic vision exists for integrating these new and existing technologies, nor how E-Nav might require changes to working methods, standards, regulations and tools. Most likely E-Nav will not cause a revolution in the way navigation is currently undertaken, but over time a more systematic and holistic approach will emerge.

Marine navigation is well behind other modes of transport (aviation and road) in terms of a coordinated and systematic approach, especially through the use of modern technological developments. This represents a good opportunity for the human factors community to become involved in this area. It is argued here that for the maritime industry as a whole to benefit from E-Nav it needs to avoid many of the negative consequences that have been found when introducing new technologies and automation in other areas (such as information overload, operator over-reliance, or operator resistance). Similarly, some overarching human factors (and indeed engineering) requirements are for the systems, tools, and procedures employed to be standardized and integrated.

We believe that there will be several key human factors issues with E-Nav:

- Ensuring operator involvement in system design
- Conducting initial and ongoing operator training to ensure familiarity and competence; Developing appropriate training methods (e.g., bridge simulators) and standards.

- Applying better standardization of bridge layouts, maritime equipment, and procedures, especially as there might be multiple suppliers involved in E-Nav.
- Engaging the whole industry in both the overall concept and the solution, and explaining ("selling") how E-Nav can be a tool to aid navigation, and providing feedback.
- Exploring maritime reduced crewing issues associated with E-Nav.
- Ensuring against inappropriate use (e.g., through independent checking).
- Developing the systems to fit the needs of the operators and the requirements of the task. Therefore, we need to make certain that the needs and potential benefits drive the E-Nav technology solution, and not vice versa.
- Considering variations between navigation operators.
- Considering how E-Nav may degrade skills/competency.
- Considering how E-Nav may influence job satisfaction.
- Integrating new E-Nav tools with existing equipment and procedures.
- Designing intuitive and usable controls and displays.
- Having appropriate change management systems to assist with the successful introduction of E-Nav.

Clearly there is plenty to keep the human factors professional busy. It is therefore essential that such E-Nav systems are properly developed, reviewed, and validated, and that they take the human element into account throughout this whole process.

6.5   Crew responses to technology

Unless a ship's HMI is ergonomically designed, the information it presents may overload or confuse the operator. For example, where it is possible for multiple warnings to occur simultaneously, these may be prioritized so that less critical or urgent warnings are not presented. As in the road environment, perhaps the greatest problem in the immediate future may be the potential information overload from the increase of unintegrated devices and systems on board. Six human factors issues that should be considered as new technologies increasingly weave their way into the maritime domain are reviewed below. These include operator workload, behavioral adaptation, loss of skills, understanding the limitations of technology, crew acceptance, and given the importance of the area, the final issue, situation awareness, is reviewed in more detail.

6.5.1   Operator workload

Physical and mental workload was introduced in Chapter 3. The focus here is on mental workload from new technologies on ships. In the near future it is likely that many maritime operators on the bridge or engine room will be exposed, sometimes simultaneously, to information from several sources:

- from crew verbal instructions
- from the environment around them (especially if in close proximity to other ships)
- from multiple instrument displays and alarms,from various crew monitoring devices (e.g., fatigue detection technologies)
- from entertainment and communication systems

Controlling workload is a key factor with new technology—too high a workload can lead to the demands exceeding an operator's capacity to cope, whereas low levels can lead to operator boredom and being "out of the control loop." In maritime operations, often a problem is that the workload is unevenly distributed, rather than simply reduced: for example, at key times (such as responding to a series of alarms in the engine room following a component failure) workload is excessively high, whereas on most occasions the technology reduces the engine room operators to passive monitoring of the system.

6.5.2 *Behavioral adaptation*

Maritime operators may adapt positively or negatively to new technologies. Positive adaptation occurs when a new technology brings about a positive change in operator behavior, such as when a new navigation system saves fuel and increases safety while being acceptable and well liked by the operators. Negative adaptation may make the operators engage in riskier behaviors (e.g., seeing how long they could remain vigilant when using fatigue detection technologies).

6.5.3 *Loss of skills*

In the longer term, removal of operators from the direct control of a ship may result in their skills and abilities declining. This is particularly a problem when they might need to identify problems and act in the case of an emergency. For example, with ECDIS, there may be a loss of traditional navigational skills among operators. Coupled to the skill fade, there may be a loss of motivation and/or status, as they may view their roles as simple monitors of equipment, rather than as skilled mariners.

6.5.4 *Understanding the limitations of the technology*

It is critical that crew understand the technical limitations of the new technologies with which they interact. If their expectations of new device's performance are inaccurate, or too high, they may expect the system to alert them to critical situations or to prevent them from having an accident in situations in which the system is not capable of doing so. Equally, as crew adapt to new systems on board, they may become over-reliant on them. For example, the earlier-mentioned grounding of the *Royal Majesty* in 1995 was in part due to over-reliance by the officers of the watch on the new automation of their bridge system—officers were lulled into false sense of security and did not realize that the vessel was several miles off course.

Training and other forms of procedural guidance need to make crew aware of the capabilities and limitations of new technologies, especially in case of emergency, or when they move to different ships. However, such training and guidance, although necessary, is not always sufficient, in that it ultimately relies on the absence of individual human error, rather than on creating safe and error-tolerant maritime systems.

6.5.5   Crew acceptance

Very little research has been undertaken into the acceptability of many of the new technologies on board ships. If crew preferences are not well understood before new ship systems are introduced, the systems may be unacceptable when deployed. Similar to the issue of usability discussed earlier, technologies that are not accepted by the operator are less likely to be used properly and are more likely to be sabotaged or misused; thus any inherent potential for increasing safety or efficiency may not be realized.

6.5.6   Technology and situation awareness

As has been repeatedly mentioned in this book, tackling human error (whether organizational or individual error) is one of the main challenges facing maritime operations today, and is an area where many benefits are likely. Here we focus on one aspect of human error: lack of situation awareness (SA). As described in Chapter 2, up to the present day, research on SA has been largely restricted to the aviation industry, and to some degree to the medical and road transport sectors. However, SA is important in any complex and dynamic environment, such as the maritime domain. Sadly, until now, few researchers have examined situation awareness in the maritime environment.

On ships it is important that crewmembers are aware of critical voyage parameters, the state of their onboard systems as a whole, their own location, and also the location of important reference points. As the mental models of each operator will vary, so each may have a unique awareness of the situation. Hence the safety of the voyage depends on the level of situational awareness that the crew is able to attain both individually and together and may be limited by the SA of the individual who has the command of the ship, usually the master or the pilot. This is of particular importance when navigating a ship near land or in restricted waterways.

In addition to the influence on SA by the characteristics and processing mechanisms of an operator (as noted in Chapter 2), many environmental and system factors also have a large impact. Each of these factors can act to seriously challenge the ability of the crew to maintain a high level of SA. Factors that have a major influence on loss of SA include workload (too low and high), system complexity, automation, safety culture, teamwork, and communication.

Situation awareness and level of technology. In research undertaken by the authors of this book (Grech, Horberry, and Smith 2002), the SA taxonomy was applied to an investigation of causal factors underlying shipping accidents, based on casualty investigation reports. Initial results revealed that by far the most prevalent casual factor was some error in the crew's SA. The study revealed that 71 percent of human errors were SA problems. Building on this, the relationship between loss of SA and the level of technology on board ships was then analyzed. It was hypothesized that one of the consequences of increasing level of technology is a loss of situation awareness, which significantly influences performance in abnormal, time-critical situations. The study linked the level of technology with the age of the ship; hence the level of technology was operationally defined by the age of the vessel. An interval period of five years was taken as the age gap that was linked to the level of technology. A strong correlation of 0.83 between loss of SA and age of the ship was obtained (with newer ships having more of a loss of SA), indicating that SA is a problem with increasing levels of technology and serious considerations are required to mitigate this.

Finally, the work provided an indication of the relative frequencies of various causal factors associated with SA errors in the maritime domain. The majority of SA errors were due to failure to monitor or observe data. In most cases these errors were due to momentary task distractions or high workload. However, high workload has also featured in other SA errors such as memory loss and misperception of data/information. If requirements are moderately excessive, there may be a measurable degradation in performance of simple, supportive tasks associated with the navigation and safe handling of the vessel, such as routine communications, watchkeeping, navigation, and engine room monitoring.

Overall the work has demonstrated that loss of SA is an important factor in many maritime accidents. Also, greater use of automation seems to be linked to a greater loss of SA. Although SA is currently a "trendy" area of research, the results have demonstrated that further work on this topic in the maritime environment is worthwhile.

6.6   Possible solutions for the maritime domain and further work in this area

From the above, it can be concluded that new developments within the maritime domain, such as single-person watchkeeping on the bridge, fully automated engine rooms, and other automated systems, will change the role of the human operators from active to passive participants in the day-to-day activity of the system. However, as discussed in this chapter there are inherent problems associated with this change. The longer operators are removed from being active participants in the system, the more likely they will lose understanding of the way it works; this is especially problematic in abnormal situations when operators are expected to solve and rectify a problem.

From a positive perspective, new maritime technology can have significant safety and efficiency benefits. Many communication and navigation systems in use today (such as IBS) could only have been dreamed about by mariners fifty years ago. The point is that technology needs to be developed and introduced from both a human-centered and a maritime need perspective; for example, considering the crew's needs of the technology and analyzing how it will be integrated with other technologies and training systems, and not purely introduced because the technology is available. Only by taking this approach will we be likely to make a significant reduction in the number of maritime accidents that are due to some aspect of human error.

The potential effect of automation on the performance of shipboard tasks and the role of advanced technology systems aimed at reducing the risk of maritime accidents has yet to be fully explored, especially with reference to new navigation systems (such as E-Nav). Although advanced technology can be viewed as beneficial in terms of being able to process more information, one of the consequences of increasing level of technology is a loss of situation awareness, which significantly influences performance in abnormal, time-critical situations. The decision to rely or not to rely on automation can be one of the most important decisions each member of the crew has to make. In some cases, crewmembers may rely too much on the automation and fail to check and monitor its performance. On the other hand, they may have lost confidence in their own activities to perform the tasks manually, which obviously defeats the purpose of automation itself. As can be learned from the aviation domain, making the automation more directly observable and capable of being modified to the exact demands of the situation (by the technology adapting to the operator, not vice versa) are possible steps forward, but a large amount of work needs to be undertaken to make this happen.

The acceptance by and acceptability to operators of new maritime equipment is an ongoing issue. If the experiences of introducing new technologies to the manufacturing or road transport domains are in any way applicable, then there might be serious issues regarding introducing new technologies if the acceptability of these devices for the operators is not measured and considered. Involving the operators at all stages from the concept through to the evaluation of a working system is the best way forward; likewise, making sure systems and technologies are introduced based on an identified need is our recommendation.

6.7 Conclusion

As with most other complex sociotechnical systems, maritime operations can be a fertile area for the human factors specialist to work in. It seems likely that future elements of the system will indeed become safer. We expect that sophisticated management systems will be increasingly employed, and new technologies will be designed and evaluated more from a human-centered perspective. Despite this, the overall physical and cognitive characteristics of operators will remain largely unchanged. Even if maritime operations become even more automated in the future, the safety specialist will still need to consider human strengths and weaknesses when designing future ship systems.

chapter seven

Organization, society and culture

7.1   Introduction

For many years, accident analyses within the maritime domain followed an individualistic approach to human error. Failures originating from "operator error" tended to dominate the main concerns of maritime accident investigators and regulators. Such methods substantially changed following the roll-on/roll-off passenger ferry *Herald of Free Enterprise* casualty. This tragedy has already been mentioned in previous chapters but due to its relevance we grant it particular attention in this chapter. On March 27, 1987 the passenger ferry *Herald of Free Enterprise* left Zeebrugge harbor in Belgium for Dover in England. Shortly after leaving harbor, water started flooding the car decks because the bow doors had been left open. The vessel listed to starboard and the ship rapidly filled with water resulting in the vessel capsizing. More than 190 people lost their lives with many others injured. At the time it was considered to be one of the worst ferry disasters to hit the European shores. Following the sinking of the *Herald of Free Enterprise,* the initial conclusion by the company's management was that the ferry sank for one simple reason: one of the crew was sleeping in the cabin and left the loading doors open. The defining moment came about following the Wreck Commissioners judgment on the causes of this tragic event. After acknowledging the shipboard errors of the crew, the commissioner indicated that the "underlying or cardinal faults lay higher up in the company" and that "from top to bottom the body corporate was infected with the disease of sloppiness" (Sheen 1987).

The *Herald of Free Enterprise* conclusion spread the view that safety stretches beyond the individual *human error* and embraces organizational factors, which in turn influence operator performance. This chapter seeks to provide a basis for understanding some aspects of maritime social and cultural attributes and look at the causes of organizational failures.

Both these elements form part of the sociotechnical system model described in Chapter 1 under Society and Culture and Organizational

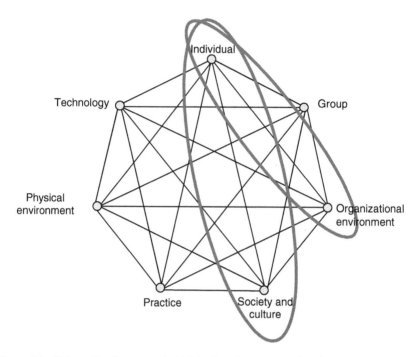

Figure 7.1 Interaction between individual and society and culture; and individual and some aspects of the organizational environment within the sociotechnical system model.

Environment. Hence, the focus of this chapter is on the interaction between individual and society and culture; and individual and some aspects of the organizational environment as illustrated in the sociotechnical system in Figure 7.1. In addition, this chapter provides some insight into current safety control strategies.

We end this chapter by also looking at the interaction between the individual and practice in the sociotechnical system.

7.2   From individual to organizational failure

7.2.1   To blame or not to blame

"Human error is viewed as the cause of accidents with humans being the main contributors to more than seventy-five percent of them." Unfortunately, this view is still expressed even today, where it is not uncommon for shipmasters and crew to be blamed and arrested by authorities immediately following shipping casualties. Such was the case in the aftermath of the oil tanker *Erika* accident. On December 12, 2000, the *Erika* broke in half off the Bay of Biscay in France, spilling most of its crude oil content, resulting in a major oil spill and causing an environmental disaster. Of course, the public demanded to know who was to blame. The authorities initially directed culpability wholly toward the shipmaster and crew. It took some time before the crewmembers were eventually released. Unfortunately this is not the only such case.

On November 27, 1997, the IMO adopted Resolution 849 to provide IMO member states with some guidance on maritime casualty investigation procedures. The heart of this IMO code actually specifies that casualty investigations should be carried out to identify contributing factors and provide recommendations *without apportioning blame or determining liability*. On the contrary, often investigations in the maritime domain conclude that people in the operational part of the system failed in their role (e.g., did not follow procedures or missed important information). It is not uncommon for final recommendations of investigations to propose retraining of individuals, or implementation of new regulations to further tighten and restrict their roles. Some accident reports imply that the individual *consciously chose* an error-prone course of action, further compounding a culture of blame and scapegoating. Dekker (2002) refers to this as the "bad apple theory." This problem becomes more serious when human error is viewed as emanating from one single source. Decker provides multiple reasons why regression to the bad apple theory occurs:

- Resource and time pressure constraints in accident investigations;
- Initial reaction to failure, which may blur judgment;
- Hindsight bias, where hindsight is confused with actual reality;
- Political interference where deeper probing into sources of failure is discouraged, limiting access to data or making certain recommendations; and
- Lack or limited human factors knowledge where investigators may not really know where or how to look for system failures.

Reasons for adherence to this blame culture may be varied. From the individual perspective, masters of ships traditionally are compelled to feel ultimately responsible for the vessel and its crew, and in most cases they expect and are expected to take the blame when things go wrong. In the case of some organizations there is considerable advantage in being able to separate individual fallibility from corporate responsibility. Furthermore, attributing liability to a single source is often seen to be more expedient and desirable. Political pressure also plays a part in this blame cycle. Public outcry may compel authorities to assign blame to people at the *operational end* of a system, as this is the more visible and easier to identify cause, as happened in the *Erika* casualty.

James Reason (1997) developed a solid and generally well accepted foundation for organizational failure theory and provides some suggestions on how to break free from this blame cycle. He provides some basic facts regarding human performance that need to be observed:

- Human actions are almost always constrained by factors beyond an individual's immediate control;
- Within a skilled, experienced, and largely well intentioned workforce, situations are more amenable to improvement than people;
- People cannot easily avoid those actions that they did not intend to perform in the first place;
- Errors have multiple causes: personal, task, situational, and organizational factors. (Reason 1997, p. 128)

The recent introduction of the International Safety Management (ISM) Code, now mandatory for most merchant ships, incorporates a philosophy similar to IMO Resolution 849, in which an environment should be created where safety is more important than punishment. Only when this philosophy is truly adopted will real progress be made in the management of safety within the maritime domain. The ISM code is described in more detail later in this chapter.

Organizational failures research has highlighted two important distinctions related to failure types. It has shown that human error is not only connected to people at the operational end of the system (active failures), but can also emanate from organizational failings (latent failures). Many researchers today view human error (Dekker 2002; Reason 1997) as emanating from *a family of problems of behavior* that originates from various sources such as poor management, inadequate supervision, and lack of communication.

7.2.2   *Active and latent failures*

This background brings us to the discussion of *active* and *latent* failures. Performance of frontline personnel is usually associated with active failures, whereas latent failures are those that lie dormant for varying periods of time (Reason 1997). The maritime domain has now started to address and look for common latent failures. The catalyst for this change was a spate of major accidents, such as the passenger ferry *Herald of Free Enterprise*. Accident investigations relating to this event and others revealed organizational shortfalls, with some lying dormant for several years prior to the actual events.

There are two main factors that distinguish between active and latent failures: (1) time and (2) the originator of failure. Active failures result in an immediate failure and these are usually committed by persons at the operational end of the system such as shipboard crew. Latent failures, on the other hand, usually exist for some time and may lie dormant for long periods (sometimes even years) prior to triggering an accident sequence of events. An important aspect of latent failures is that they arise from high-level decisions made by, for example, regulators or ship management companies. In most cases latent failures provide the conditions for active failures to occur. Studies of major accidents have shown that errors almost always arise from a combination of both active and latent failures.

For the most part, active failures on their own do not lead to any major consequences as they are usually captured by the system defenses and safeguards or are managed by the crew. However, these may sometimes surpass system defenses and safeguards and result in an incident or accident. This happened in the *Herald of Free Enterprise* where the causes for this accident have been traced to latent conditions deeply rooted in the system.

The assistant bosun on the *Herald of Free Enterprise* whose duty was to close the bow doors (which were left open) was sleeping in his cabin. The system defenses had failed to detect and correct this. The senior bosun who was close by and knew about this did not take action to close the bow doors. He considered this not to be his duty at the time. The duty chief mate, the last line of defense in the closure of the bow doors, assumed that everything was in order without visually verifying this. He saw a man standing around the bow doors from a distance and assumed it was the assistant bosun about to close the doors. His message to the master was that the bow doors had been closed when in fact they were not.

Another factor that would have assisted in this line of defense is bow door indicators. In this regard the captain had asked for bow and stern door remote indication (e.g., closed-circuit television) several times before; however, this request had always been refused by top management. It is also probable that the crew did not deviate too much from their usual practices (allowed by the organization) prior to the accident, which led to a *drift into failure* mode contributing to the slow degradation and final breaking-up of the sociotechnical system. For example, the ship management company permitted and tolerated overloading (excessive freight weights and numbers of passengers). So overloading of the vessel was a common occurrence. The company also allowed use of demanding shipboard work schedules with excessive working hours (the assistant bosun was on duty for a long time prior to dozing off in his cabin).

Another aspect was the very unstable roll-on/roll-off design of this vessel. On this particular occasion these weaknesses combined with other active and latent conditions, which finally aligned in such a way as to create the conditions that led to this tragic event. An easy way to illustrate this is via Reason's (1997) *Swiss cheese* model as shown in Figure 7.2. This analogy shows the breach of system defenses caused by both latent conditions inherent within the system and active failures. The breach is shown by holes in the system defenses. Usually the layers of defenses interact and support one another. However, in some instances the holes may align in such a way as to create an *accident trajectory* such as happened in the *Herald of Free Enterprise*. The bosun sleeping in his cabin played a part in the active failure. The chief mate failed in his role as one of the system's important line of defenses, by not visually verifying the closure of bow doors. This omission played a significant role in this accident. These holes also came about from latent conditions present in the system, further weakening the defenses. One of these was the poor design of the *Herald of Free Enterprise,* such that it was prone

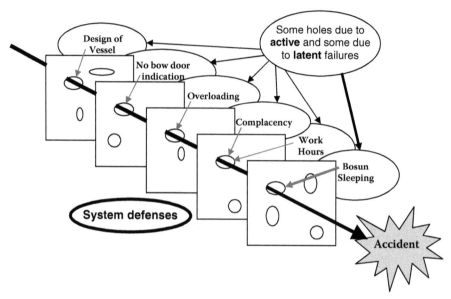

Figure 7.2 The *Swiss cheese* model showing the accident path aligning through the breached defenses created by active and latent failures represented as *holes* in the system. Adapted with permission of Reason (1997).

to capsizing when large quantities of water swept the car deck. Finally, the combination of active failures (in this case crew inaction) and latent conditions (ship design and refusal to fit warnings by the organization) resulted in this disastrous outcome.

7.2.3   Drift into failure

The drift into failure mode mentioned in the previous section is an important concept that warrants a bit more insight here. In this regard, Dekker (2005) describes how accidents can be considered the outcome of an entire system breaking down after "a long period" of degradation rather than the outcome of single events (e.g., actions of single persons) linked together in causal chains. This is what we mean when we refer to a drift into failure. It is important to understand that this degradation happens slowly over a long period of time. Dekker claims that the drift into failure approach can be used to understand accidents where no immediate failure can be found. An example he uses to illustrate drift into failure is the Alaska Airlines flight 261 crash which occurred in 2000. The cause of the crash was related to the maintenance interval of the horizontal stabilizer of the airplane, which slowly "degraded" over a period of four decades (1960s to 2000) that the aircraft was in service, until it crashed. The maintenance interval for that specific part was carried out in accordance with the original manufacturer's procedures, developed when the aircraft was initially launched in the 1960s. The procedures stated a maintenance interval of 300 to 350 flying hours for the horizontal stabilizer of the aircraft. Over time, this interval slowly increased due to various reasons, one of which was commercial pressure. In 2000 this maintenance interval period grew to be more than 5,000 flying hours. This finally led to the system to breakdown leading to the accident.

7.3   Culture in the maritime work environment

As a follow-up to the topic of social role and power discussed in Chapter 4, this section looks at culture in the maritime work environment and discusses the way culture affects our work environment. Culture has been described as the shared way of life, within a group of people, an organization, a profession, or a nation. It incorporates norms, attitudes, values, and practices that these groups might share. Culture affects the way people communicate, make decisions, and evaluate risks. Helmreich and Merritt (2004) present three types of culture that can influence the work environment:

1. National
2. Professional
3. Organizational

These types of culture have an influence on individual attitudes, values, and team interactions and can lead to both positive and negative human performance on board ships, such as happened in the *Herald of Free Enterprise* where a negative culture prevailed.

7.3.1   National culture

National culture plays a strong role in shaping attitudes and behavior. In today's world, merchant shipping is indeed considered one of the most international of industries. Therefore, various national cultures exist and interact. As indicated in Chapter 1, it is not uncommon to have a ship managed in one country, registered in a second country, classed in a third country, and crewed by people from multiple countries. This creates a situation where organizations and people from diverse national cultures need to interact, and this presents some interesting challenges for the maritime domain. Factors such as communication, teamwork, responsibility, and authority may all differ culturally. This may create some problems as indicated in Chapter 4. For example, some countries may use a more direct way of communication than others, which may perhaps sound rude to other cultures. In some countries it may be perceived as offensive or impolite to question higher authority whereas in other countries this may not be the case. These and other factors may lead to potential misunderstandings and conflict in cross-cultural encounters.

7.3.2   *Professional culture*

Professional culture concerns attributes of the profession and includes such factors as traditions of profession, training processes, associated risks, and responsibilities, as well as characteristics of persons making up the profession. Compared to other professions such as aviation, seafaring is an old tradition. For this reason, merchant shipping possesses a strong professional culture. As indicated in Chapter 3, crewmembers not only work on a ship but also live there and sometimes this can extend over long periods of time. This leads to lack of social contact with family and friends and creates to some extent an independent and isolated institution. There is a tightly scheduled daily routine on board, with the whole schedule enforced by a set of rules from a higher authority.

Another important aspect related to professional culture is socialization. There was a time when the recruitment process selected people to join the seafaring profession based on certain social characteristics. This ensured effective membership of the organization, with the amount of socialization (the learning of values and norms) required very small. Today, however, with an ever-shrinking pool of applicants wanting to work at sea, organizations are almost compelled to accept any applicant that comes along, which results in greater amounts of socialization required in order to attain the desired level of social characterization.

There also exists, to some extent, a *social* and *power distance* between the ordinary sailors and the officers. Power distance is related to the way people perceive differences in their status with respect to their subordinates or even colleagues. Officers, for example, have the power to discipline any ordinary sailor. In addition, the authority of the captain is absolute on board a ship. Perhaps because of its old tradition the maritime domain has to some degree been slow in embracing such concepts as open communication and teamwork. Such practices are now universal in domains such as the aviation. Fortunately, professional culture is dynamic rather than static. This means that circumstances or interventions such as training practices like crew resource management (CRM) and bridge team management courses, as indicated in Chapter 4 and which are discussed later in this chapter, can change established norms and values. However, change in professional culture requires both a level of strong intervention and a large amount of time.

7.3.3   *Organizational culture*

Organizational culture and practices have been found to influence individual attitudes and behaviors toward work. Similar to national culture, organizations also develop norms, values, and beliefs that are reflected in the strategies and attitudes of management toward such aspects as open communication, teamwork, and training. Some accidents can be traced to organizational policies and decisions, which can lead to human error types such as lack of situation awareness, high fatigue, and unacceptable workload levels, with serious potential implications, as discussed in Chapter 3. The maritime domain has only very recently started addressing the influence of organizational culture on crew behavior. One such initiative in this area is the Man/Ship Interface System (MASIS) project (European Commission 1998). This project aimed to assess practical tools and procedures capable of reducing the impact of human error in shipping. One of the main contributing factors identified as affecting human behavior on board ships is the interaction between human(s) and organization(s).

Organizational influences on human behavior have reached an advanced stage of maturity in other high-risk industries, such as the aviation domain, with a number of models developed to reflect this. For example, Shappell and Wiegmann (2000) developed a Human Factors Analyses and Classification System (HFACS) model based on the active/latent failure principle, which has been applied in the aviation domain. The framework is based on Reason's Swiss cheese model and looks at a number of dimensions down the chain of events leading to system failures. This model identifies a number of organizational factors as influencing human behavior: (1) resource management; (2) organizational climate; and (3) organizational processes. We have, in Chapter 1, also described the SHEL model and the ECCAIRS Explanatory Factors taxonomy framework. From these, the sociotechnical system model was developed, specifically customized for use within the maritime domain. The sociotechnical system model, described in Chapter 1, provides a more systematic approach for viewing human factors and incorporates the society and culture and organizational environment interaction factors, which are the focus of this chapter.

7.3.3.1 From organizational culture to safety culture

In this section we have described how three cultures, professional, national, and organizational, influence attitudes and behaviors at work. It is only if the effect of culture on individual operator behavior is not acknowledged that it could potentially lead to more serious problems. Hence, without proper attention and training, this trend toward diversity of cultures can develop into many human behavioral problems, which can lead to low motivation and performance during maritime operations. As shown in Figure 7.3, it is ultimately the organizational culture that channels the effects of national and professional cultures into shaping attitudes and behavior toward safety and performance. Hence, even with the most appropriate regulations, best-designed equipment, and the most-qualified and well-trained personnel, generally systems are not better or safer than the system or organization that bounds them. Individual behavior is therefore influenced by the organization, and one means of inducing optimum behavior is to develop a good safety culture.

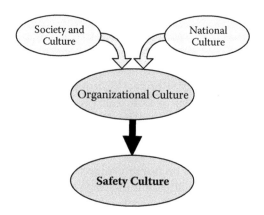

Figure 7.3 The interaction and influence of national, professional, and organizational cultures on safety culture.

7.3.4   Safety culture

Safety is not an easy concept to define as it incorporates many dimensions; however, it would be appropriate to state that safety is a characteristic of a system that strives for incident- and injury-free operations and does not permit unacceptable risks to be taken. A simple and somewhat attractive notion is to equate a good safety culture with a low rate of accidents. Although it can be argued that an organization with a good safety culture might be expected to have a low accident rate, the reverse is not necessarily true. Organizations with a poor safety culture may indeed be simply lucky and have low numbers of accidents. Within this context, safety culture deals with the extent to which people and groups within an organization strive to improve and communicate safety concerns and are willing to continuously learn, adapt, and modify behavior based on lessons learned. A submission by the United Kingdom to the IMO Maritime Safety Committee in 2003 defines safety culture as "a culture in which there is considerable informed endeavour to reduce risks to the individual, ships and the marine environment to a level that is as low as is reasonably practicable" (International Maritime Organization 2003).

Westrum (1992) developed a concept for distinguishing between various organizational safety cultures. Other leading researchers in this field continued building on this concept linking this organizational evolution to safety culture. As shown in Figure 7.4 organizations undergo a series of evolutions in the way they respond to safety culture starting from *pathological* to *generative*. An organization, therefore, moves from an unsafe to a safe system state and only after reaching a certain level in the evolutionary process can an organization be said to take safety seriously enough to have a safety culture. Unsafe, *pathological* organizations exhibit blame tendencies, where errors and mistakes are dismissed or even hidden, and where

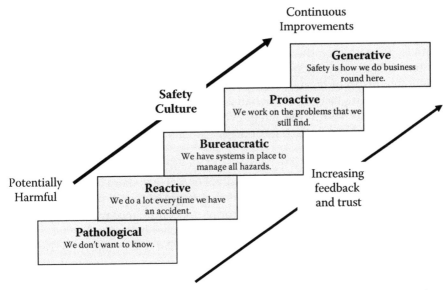

Figure 7.4   The various levels of an organizational evolution and its links to safety culture. Adapted from Hudson (2001) and Westrum (1992).

feedback and new ideas are usually discouraged. It is fairly obvious that pathological organizations are not interested in safety. A *reactive* organization, the next stage in the safety cultural evolution, is one in which safety issues begin to acquire some importance. This is often driven by both internal and external factors, perhaps as a result of having many incidents and accidents. Reactive organizations have a lower accident prevention capability than *bureaucratic* organizations, which is the next stage in the evolution. At this stage in the evolution, risks and safety defenses are reviewed after an accident has occurred rather than before. In bureaucratic organizations quantitative risk assessment techniques and cost–benefit analyses are used to justify safety and to measure its effectiveness, although to some extent new ideas are seen as presenting problems. At this stage, despite what can become an impressive safety record, safety is still seen as an add-on. As the name implies *proactive* organizations incorporate more proactive approaches to safety, such as training and safety management systems. However, proactive organizations lack the ability to *learn* from concrete evidence collected after an actual accident has taken place. Finally, *generative* organizations fully integrate safe behavior into everything the organization does. They also make good use of information, observations, and new ideas captured within the system. One crucial difference between this final stage and prior stages is that the human factor is considered to include both the individual and the organization.

Marshall (2006) notes that the challenges involved in moving from a pathological to a generative state involves "a stated commitment from the board and the executive management of the organization. They must not only be receptive, they must also demonstrate their commitment through the active support of the safety management system and in the adoption of safety initiatives. Importantly, the organization must move from a blame culture to a 'just' culture. A just culture recognises that errors and mistakes are the inevitable result of human failings and that systemic deficiencies are often key contributing factors" (Marshall 2006). Once an organization reaches the generative state within the safety evolution it will face many challenges to remain at that level. In fact, most organizations shift up and down between the various levels.

There has been a growing interest in recent years within the maritime domain in the concept of safety culture. For starters, there has partly been a shift away from the behavioral factors that might be responsible for accidents and incidents, such as individual error or noncompliance with safety procedures, toward organizational factors that influence behavior. The term *safety culture* has been discussed in detail in the *Herald of Free Enterprise* casualty report. The report indicated that crew behavior had a detrimental effect on the final outcome. Successive enquiries into this casualty indicated that crew behavior that led to negative outcomes came about from a poor safety culture within the organization, which included among others poor communication, unclear job responsibilities, and management failures. It is therefore of no surprise that organizations with a poor track record, lack of or poor implementation of regulations, and a lack of quality control and training may experience an increase in the likelihood of a system failure due to the greater number of malfunctions that can interact, such as what happened in the *Herald of Free Enterprise*.

Some industries have developed widely varying techniques for addressing the uncertainties arising from human involvement, with varying degrees of success. The aviation domain, for example, has been particularly successful in this regard, with the adoption of a nonpunitive approach, ensuring that safety data on errors is collected in order to identify where improvements need to be made. The importance of data collection for managing safety is discussed in more detail in Chapter 8. Within this context, an evaluation of the working environments of the maritime and the aviation domains was carried out by one of the authors with the aim of identifying differences and similarities in their safety culture. This evaluation is shown in Table 7.1, where information was obtained following a literature review and short interviews with subject matter experts. This short review allows us to draw some parallels and distinctions between social organizations within aviation and the maritime domain in order to understand how safety culture might influence safety-critical behaviors. Looking at best practice from other sectors can serve to inform the sorts of successful strategies that are effective in other domains, which can then be used in the maritime domain, and vice versa. This review was conducted from a macro level perspective, and was not intended to be a comprehensive study. The review includes

Table 7.1 A Review of Safety Culture of the Maritime and Aviation Domain Using the IACO (1992) Safety Culture Dimensions

	Maritime	Aviation
Willingness by senior staff to accept criticism and open views	Ships have always been socially organized into a strict hierarchical pyramid with the master at the top through the officers to the crew at the base. Aboard the ship the master has command. This authoritarian role, thought to be functional for ship emergencies, is definitely dysfunctional for inter-ship/shore emergencies.	Part of CRM training. Generally crew must be in agreement. They are trained to check each other's actions and to be assertive if they feel that one or other has made an error. Decision making based on goal hierarchy.
Importance of communicating relevant safety information	In 1998, the ISM Code became mandatory for some merchant ship types. It establishes safety management objectives and requires a safety management system to be in place. However, recent studies indicate that the ISM may not guarantee proof of adequate system safety.	High priority. ATC needs to communicate effectively to pilots. Tightly circumscribed vocabulary and set of commands that controllers and pilots are permitted to use.
Educated and trained staff in understanding the consequences of human error	There is a general lack of understanding in identifying, developing, and implementing effective measures to prevent specific human error problems that dominate casualties within the maritime domain. This can be seen in the lack of or poor incident reporting procedures.	Part of training curriculum and training is a mandatory licensing requirement by the ICAO. Gained wide acceptance in aviation and seen as a valuable tool. Part of CRM training, which focuses on effective crew coordination, communication, and human factors.

Table 7.1 A Review of Safety Culture of the Maritime and Aviation Domain Using the IACO (1992) Safety Culture Dimensions (Continued)

	Maritime	Aviation
Understanding of workplace hazards by staff members	Generally a good understanding. However, potential risks of hazards due to a decrement in cognitive functions (human error) not well proliferated within the maritime domain. There is a culture to continue working irrespective of cognitive limitations. In addition, economic pressures are enormous and demands to meet schedules often result in increased levels of high-risk behavior. Also potential variances exist between and within national cultures that influence how risk and safety are perceived and managed. Culturally this domain has a high-risk perception tendency.	Generally a good understanding. Risk assessment and analyses models used for safety assessments. Standards set by ICAO are based on risk analyses modeling. Generally a proactive industry. Will not violate standard procedures. Trained not to take risks. Pilot decision-making training introduced in some countries, which trains on attitudes and behavior.
Promotion of realistic and workable safety rules	Lack of uniformity in approaches within the maritime domain makes it difficult to control and regulate the management of risk. This could be less of a problem on naval vessels.	Checklists are regularly used. Designed to be followed precisely. Adherence is seen as imperative for safe flight. ATC is highly proceduralized.

subcomponents of safety culture as defined by the International Civil Aviation Organization (ICAO 1992):

- Senior management's willingness to accept criticism and openness to opposing views;
- The importance of communicating relevant safety information;
- Level of staff training and education in understanding the consequences of unsafe acts;
- Staff's understanding of hazards within the workplace; and
- Promotion of realistic and workable safety rules.

Table 7.1 demonstrates that human factors is well understood in some industries, such as aviation, but is perhaps not that well understood or applied in the maritime domain. Within the maritime domain there has been little work done in trying to understand the effects of organizational culture on safe and efficient performance. Nevertheless, the picture is not that bleak, as considerable progress has been made in the area of safety and error management within the maritime domain, which is described in more detail in the next sections. One step in the right direction is the U.K. submission to the IMO Maritime Safety Committee in 2003 mentioned above. This provides a number of key characteristics that need to be considered for achieving a proactive maritime safety culture conveyed in Table 7.2.

7.3.5 Safety control strategies

An important function of organizations and their crews is to ensure that they have adequate defenses in place, first to avoid errors, and second to trap and manage errors when they cannot be avoided. In addition, a robust recovery process within the system, such as a person to detect the error and initiate action, would likely lead to recovery before safety of the system is compromised. On the other hand, if crewmembers miss or exacerbate errors, an unsafe system state is likely to result. The more effective the error management and recovery process, the less likely system failures will result. Hence, the need for a more proactive approach to human and organizational error is crucial.

In road safety, countermeasures are usually categorized as falling under one of the three Es. Although this principle has not been generally applied to the maritime environment, it is certainly possible. These are:

1. *Engineering*—for example, designing more accident-tolerant ships.
2. *Education and Training*—for example, through licensing and ongoing publicity campaigns to warn of specific dangers, such as fatigue and fitness for duty for operators.
3. *Enforcement*—both to act as a deterrent and to potentially remove repeated offenders from the maritime system (e.g., having a strict drug policy, and preventing offenders being re-employed in other maritime operations).

It must be noted that these three areas are not mutually exclusive—they may all be used to address a major maritime safety issue. In general terms the three Es have been used successfully in some areas of transport safety; however, they often serve purely as a broad framework in which to initiate action, rather than as a formula to develop detailed countermeasures. One strategy that can be categorized under education and training within the three Es and is increasingly being adopted within the maritime domain as indicated in Chapter 4 is CRM training. Other formalized control strategies adopted are Safety Management Systems, which incorporate the use of

Table 7.2 The U.K. Submission to the IMO Maritime Safety Committee (2003) on Key Characteristics Recommended for Achieving a Proactive Maritime Safety Culture

Stakeholder participation	Ensure that all stakeholders concerned with the identification, assessment, and management of safety-related risks are involved in determining the appropriateness and effectiveness of measures employed to mitigate these risks
Commitment and visibility	Ensure that all those responsible for managing risks show commitment to the development and support of a safety culture
Productivity/safety relationship	Ensure that the principles of a proactive safety culture are recognized (this deals with concept of safety cost versus accident cost)
Trust	Ensure a pull away from a culture of compliance and strive more toward a culture of responsibility
Shared perceptions	Ensure that those managing safety-related risks have the same perception of risks as those who are exposed to them
Communication	Ensure that intentions about what are safe and unsafe practices are communicated to all stakeholders
Organizational learning	Ensure promotion of an open and honest environment with a nonpunitive approach with visible support from senior management (this needs to gain the belief of the seafarer that such a system exists)
Safety resources	Ensure that enough resources are made available to support, nurture, and develop a safety culture
Industrial relations and job satisfaction	Ensure good industrial relations exist between employee and employer, and the individuals have job satisfaction
Training	Ensure that the intrinsic relationships between training, competence, and procedures are well recognized

procedures, job aids, and warnings systems. All these factors are discussed in the next sections.

7.3.5.1 Safety management systems

Safety management systems are integrated collections of work procedures and practices used to examine and improve an organization's safety and health. Safety culture is, of course, closely linked to the philosophy underlying safety management systems.

As pointed out in Chapter 1, on July 1, 1998 the maritime domain adopted a safety management system more commonly referred to as the International Safety Management (ISM) Code. This was made mandatory by incorporating it into the IMO International Convention for the Safety of Life at Sea (SOLAS) 1974, as a new chapter.

It would be wrong to assume that the entire shipping industry did not have good safety systems in place before the ISM Code became a statutory requirement. The earliest usage of safety management systems dates to the late 1980s when some ship managers recognized the potential benefits to be derived from implementing formal management disciplines designed to enhance the safety of ship operations. The origins of the ISM Code can be traced to the late 1980s when concern was growing about poor management practices in the shipping industry. Investigations of some accidents revealed major errors on the part of management, and in 1987 guidelines were developed by IMO concerning shipboard and shore-based management to better ensure safe operation, initially for roll-on/roll-off (ro-ro) passenger ferries. This resolution actually referred to the loss of the passenger ferry *Herald of Free Enterprise,* pointing out that "the great majority of maritime accidents are due to human error and fallibility and that the safety of ships will be greatly enhanced by the establishment of improved operating practices."

The ISM Code has had a major impact, causing shipping companies to make considerable changes to their company structures and to their approach to safety culture within the industry. The ISM Code emphasizes the role of sound management in safety and pollution prevention, and establishes a number of safety management objectives:

- provision for safe practices in ship operation and a safe working environment;
- establishment of safeguards against all identified risks;
- continuous improvement in safety management skills of personnel, including preparing for emergencies.

The ISM Code requires a safety management system to be established by "the company," which can be the ship owner, ship manager, or charterer, whoever assumes responsibility for operating the ship. The company is certificated by the flag state of the ship. In the majority of cases, this certification will actually be carried out by an *approved* classification society. Its implementation is usually policed by both flag state and port state controls, who may request to verify that the necessary documentation and certification are in place and that they are being applied on board competently.

The ISM Code is widely regarded as one of the most important measures adopted by the IMO; the question of whether or not it is working as it was intended is, however, still debatable. To facilitate auditing, the ISM Code is heavily dependent on standardized processes and procedures, documentation, and audit trails. So although it is easy enough to establish whether a shipping organization is complying with the ISM Code, it does not necessarily allow an auditor to establish whether the system is as effective as it should be. A survey undertaken by Phil Anderson in 2002 on the viewpoint of ship officers on the overall success of the implementation of the ISM Code revealed some interesting findings. Some of the findings alluded to such complaints as "too much paperwork," "too many forms to fill," "too many manuals," "not enough time," "not enough people," "no support from company," "no confidence in junior officers," "safety management system is alien to the company," and "just a paperwork exercise." The study also revealed that many individuals and organizations were struggling to make the ISM work as it was intended.

It also became clear that ship operators varied in their motivation to comply with the ISM Code. Some recognized the potential benefits of a proper implementation of a good safety management system and looked at it as a way to improve their business by reducing accidents and other losses, improve efficiency, increase motivation among personnel, and improve market reputation and hence profits. Other companies were motivated by the fact that noncompliance seriously jeopardized their defenses, exposing them to claims that may be brought against them or may even prejudice their insurance coverage. Some other companies viewed compliance as a way to ensure that individuals within the company, in particular the most senior management, are not personally exposed to fines, imprisonment, or corporate manslaughter in the event of an accident, while others looked at it as a mandatory requirement leaving them with no other option. So while many companies, ships, and individuals may have experienced (and still do experience) difficulties with its implementation, there is some evidence to indicate that the ISM Code does work and the potential rewards may be worthwhile. Nevertheless, the ISM Code is not the end point as there are some important issues that the maritime research community must strive to achieve with the support of the shipping community to provide insight into where safety improvements should focus. One of these is to establish behavioral markers that can be used to measure system safety effectiveness. Methodological issues in this area are discussed in more detail in Chapter 8.

7.3.5.2   Crew resource management

Bridge resource management (as referred to in the maritime domain and mentioned in Chapter 4), is an offshoot of CRM training. CRM began in the 1970s in the aviation industry when it was recognized that many aircraft incidents were due to human error, rather than technical aspects of flying. Examples of these errors were failures of team coordination, communication, leadership, or decision making. The maritime domain absorbed the CRM philosophy after recognizing the need for nontechnical or resource management skills following a number of accidents. One example of a maritime accident in which lack of team communication and coordination was evident was on the passenger ro-ro ferry *P&OSL Aquitaine* mentioned in Chapter 6, which led to the vessel striking the berth (Marine Accident Investigation Branch 2001b). On April 27, 2000, the passenger ferry *P&OSL Aquitaine* left Dover, bound for Calais, France, with 1,241 passengers and 123 crew on board. During the first minutes while still maneuvering out of Dover, the port controllable pitch propeller (CPP) stand-by pump cut in on several occasions. This usually occurs as a result of inadequate pressure in the main CPP pump. The engineers checked the system and found nothing out of the ordinary. At this stage the chief engineer assumed that the stand-by pump was cutting in, possibly because air had entered the system following some maintenance work that was carried out previously. He expected this air to eventually vent out and the system to return to normal operation. As he thought this to be only a minor problem, he decided not to inform the master about this. Nevertheless, it was decided that during the crossing the system would continue to be monitored. While entering the port of Calais the master decided to reduce speed by pulling the controls of the CPP to astern pitch for both propellers. However, only the starboard propeller responded to the command. Unknown to the engine room and bridge teams, control of the port CPP was lost as the vessel entered Calais. On its approach to the berth in Calais, the master was unable to properly control the vessel for docking; consequently the vessel struck the berth at a speed of about seven knots. At the time of impact, many passengers were standing up ready to disembark, while others were making their way down the car deck. This resulted in many injured passengers, and both the berth and the vessel sustained heavy damage.

In this accident the master was not aware that the engineers had experienced problems with the CPP. The engineers traced what they thought to be the fault and were confident that should it reappear, it would not have an adverse effect on the performance of the propulsion plant. In view of this they did not think it was necessary to inform the master, although procedures were in place to ensure that any problems existing in the engine room that may jeopardize safe navigation had to be reported to the master before leaving port. Had the master been aware that the engineers had recently experienced problems with the CPP system, it is possible that he would have suspected that the maneuvering difficulties were related to this and possibly averted the accident. This accident provides a good example of the importance of good communication and teamwork on board a ship and highlights the overall value of CRM training.

CRM training attempts to provide a set of countermeasures against human error, as in the *P&OSL Aquitaine* example. It is based on the premise that human error is "ubiquitous and inevitable," but that "management of process" can reduce it to acceptable levels (Helmreich and Merritt 2004). CRM training helps the crew gain greater influence over the human and situational factors that contribute to critical incidents. This can help optimize the benefits of multiperson crews to significantly improve safety. Based on this, CRM training often involves:

- Leadership and teambuilding
- Time and task management
- State of the ship
- Crew attitudes and behaviors
- Effective communication
- Problem solving and decision making
- Conflict resolution
- Automation awareness
- Stress and fatigue
- Crew individual differences

Although CRM training has now become well established in the maritime curricula, as with civil aviation, there remains a question mark about how effective such training is in improving safety performance. The aviation domain has not remained static in this regard, and is now in its fifth-generation program of CRM training. They have developed sound and tested theories, methods, principles, approaches and have made content available to shape the design and delivery of CRM training. The concept of CRM has also become more diversified. For example, the notion of *resource* in the aviation domain has gone past its initial reductionist meaning and encompasses all resources, that is, not only the crew, but also the plane (and its functions), procedures, air traffic control (ATC), ground staff, and other aviation stakeholders. In the aviation domain resource management has also spread its wings to incorporate skills aspects, which go beyond the collective and interactive dimensions of the activity, and includes, among others, all individual cognitive aspects (Helmreich and Merritt 2004). Thus, CRM training deals more and more systematically—at the individual as well as the collective level—with such topics as understanding and awareness of the situation, decision making, error management, and confidence. In addition, the aviation domain has gone one step farther by introducing a variety of performance indicators such as surveys, attitude questionnaires, behavioral checklists, and confidential reports, to obtain feedback and information to guide the design of CRM training to better reflect relevant operational situations. Hence, much can be learned from the aviation industry where CRM training is concerned. Where formal evaluations of the effectiveness of such training have been undertaken, they have generally been positive. Therefore, making such training mandatory in the maritime domain would be a valuable goal for the near future.

7.3.5.3   *Procedures and job aids*

Many organizations require procedures and job aids to guide human actions when interacting with equipment, and serve as the final authority for the conduct of safe operations. The use of written forms of expression such as procedures and checklists is intended to provide information essential to the proper functioning of the ship, and to ensure the exchange of information between the crewmembers. Procedures also help to standardize operations across the organization. In most cases good written documentation and well-drafted visual procedures have also been shown to be excellent tools for crew training. Lack of written procedures or badly written procedures have the potential to result in incidents and accidents, such as what happened on the *P&OSL Aquitaine* passenger ferry accident described previously. Prior to the accident, and after the CPP stand-by pump started to cut in, the engineers decided to review the schematic and physical plans of the CPP system to fault-diagnose the problem. The drawings were in English, but the operation and maintenance manual were written in Flemish, a language that none of the engineers understood. In addition, although it had a section describing the general arrangement of the hydraulic system and function of system components, albeit written in Flemish, there was no fault-finding or troubleshooting section. This was an important omission. The third and second engineers' knowledge and experience of the system were important assets in their attempts to find out what was wrong. An operations and maintenance manual, carefully designed, easily understood, and relevant to the needs of the engineers, would have helped their thinking, and would have helped to solve the problem. There is no point in having an instruction manual if nobody can understand or use it. When it took over the vessel twelve months earlier, the management should have made sure that the CPP system manual was in a usable form (Marine Accident Investigation Branch 2001b). It is perhaps likely that this accident could have been avoided if well-written and understandable procedures and instructions were available to the engineers.

Several important aspects need to be considered in the design of procedures and job aids:

- Take a traditional human factors perspective, and ensure that procedures correspond to the way the job is actually done, by involving end users of the system in their development. In this regard if users do not understand the underlying reasoning behind a procedure or job aid, they may carry out alternative actions that appear to achieve the same purpose but are easier to perform.
- Ensure the information contained is correct and is in a usable form for the particular job/task.
- Ensure there is a distinction made between procedures used to perform the task and procedures used as regulatory standards, commonly referred to as rules.

This last point is crucial as sometimes this can lead to confusion regarding whether some procedures are actually flexible enough to allow an alternative course of actions without violating rules. The IMO, for example, has established rules and regulations governing safety and pollution prevention for use in maritime operations. Some of these rules are added and implemented as a result of findings in major casualties. *Procedure*, for example, is actually the most often used word in the ISM Code. The points of the ISM Code relating to procedures include:

- drafting all the operational procedures for the ship to perform its mission, within the context of the company's policy for safety and environmental protection;
- preparation and maintenance of operational action plans, which enable personnel to face and manage all foreseeable situations that may affect the safety of personnel or result in a pollution risk;
- systematic organization of documented internal audits on the application of procedures recommended by the company, and the follow-up of any corrective measures in line with the ISM Code;
- analysis and handling of nonconformities observed during audits and controls.

Reason (1997) has some reservations on the process of continually amending, adding, and updating rules and procedures. He states that "over time, these additions to the 'rule book' are becoming increasingly restrictive, often reducing the range of permitted actions to far less than those necessary to get the job done under anything but optimal conditions" (p. 49). What he implies here is that these rules and procedures may in time shrink and restrict allowable human actions resulting in less tolerance available to operators to carry out their work. Reason represents this in a model framework shown in Figure 7.5. So although the principle behind the introduction of new rules and procedures is to guide human behavior to safe and productive pathways, the increasing rule book may do so at the expense of restricting flexibility in the way tasks are conducted. Within this context operators should be allowed to retain sufficient authority and flexibility to permit them to bypass the procedures if they believe that circumstance warrants it.

7.3.5.4   *Procedural and adaptive training*

The environment in which crewmembers operate requires the use of procedures to allow them to respond quickly to familiar situations or routines. However, in many cases they also need to be able to respond to novel and unfamiliar situations, especially if the system does not perform as expected. In this case it is not possible to predict all the potential situations that operators will face. In some cases the very nature of a threat situation dictates that standard procedures may not be appropriate and may lead to an incorrect response, as depicted in Figure 7.5. These limitations imply that the crewmembers have to understand and then manage the threat event through their own knowledge and abilities. In terms of the "skills, rules, and knowledge" based levels of task performance introduced in Chapter 2 and commonly used in human factors work, this management of an unexpected situation would correspond to the knowledge-based stage, where automated skills or

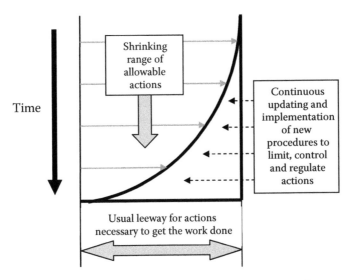

Figure 7.5   Effect of additional rules and procedures on tolerance of actions required to perform tasks. Adapted with permission from Reason (1997).

simple rules are insufficient. Training that exists for these kinds of abilities are commonly referred to as error management training, which deals specially with decision making in novel situations. Some methods to help in this are discussed further in Chapter 8. The introduction of flexible and adaptive skills, together with systematic training to handle abnormal conditions, is important so that situations are well understood, controlled, and recovered from under normal and emergency conditions.

Recent awareness of the importance of error management strategies has sparked a number of studies looking at the way people recover from incidents and near misses. Some of these studies propose that descriptions of errors, plus the methods used by crew to recover from these errors, are required to develop sound error management strategies. Training crew in threat and error management strategies also enhances the process of acquiring good situation awareness, which is crucial for increasing comprehension of a critical situation as noted in Chapter 2 and Chapter 6. This is especially important to allow for prompt and appropriate action in an emergency situation.

7.3.5.5   Warnings
The topic on warnings is discussed very briefly here, and only within the context of safety management, as this topic has already been covered more extensively in Chapter 6.

To improve system safety all hazards need to be controlled and managed. Some strategies applied to the control of maritime-related hazards include elimination/reduction of the hazard, isolation of hazard, use of engineering controls, application of administrative controls, use of personal protective equipment, and application of behavioral methods (e.g., disciplining operators). One taxonomy developed to categorize these control options is the safety* control hierarchy. Many variants of this taxonomy exist, but perhaps the simplest version has just three levels. In order of effectiveness they are:

1. *Remove the problem*—by designing it out. This might involve design of the ship, so that the hazard is not present on the ship.
2. *Place a barrier around the object*—to stop the problem from occurring by placing a barrier (physical, organizational, or temporal) around the hazard. This might include a physical guard to protect against accidental contact, or an organizational guard, where only supervised personnel work near that equipment.
3. *Implement warnings*—to provide information needed to function safely in a working environment. For example, placing notices near the equipment to indicate a hazard or having audible alarms in place in case of component or system failure.

The different levels of the hierarchy represent different levels of effectiveness. For example, *implement warnings* is placed as the very last in the safety hierarchy, behind design and guards. The reason for this is that people may not see or hear warnings, they may fail to understand the warnings, or they may not be motivated enough to pay attention or comply with warnings. Therefore, controlling the hazard at the "highest" level possible is generally seen as the most effective. However, such concerns are not a basis for not using warnings. To summarize, warnings on board ships play a specific role in assisting the crew in ensuring a level of safely is maintained.

7.4   Maintenance failures

An important issue, which has featured in several maritime accidents and falls under organizational or latent failure conditions, is ship maintenance. Maintenance failures provide the fuel for operational errors, which could set an accident sequence in motion. On board ships, maintenance tasks sometimes need to be conducted under poor physical environmental conditions. As specified in Chapter 5, these environmental conditions can affect human performance negatively, which can lead to maintenance errors or omissions being made. In some cases personnel responsible for maintenance may not be adequately trained, sometimes they take shortcuts, and sometimes they suffer slips and lapses. It is sometimes difficult to distinguish between these causes; however, more often than not, more than one cause may have been at work. What is certain, however, is that the way maintenance tasks are carried out can be a reflection of the organization's safety culture.

---

* Also referred to as hazard control hierarchy.

One shipboard example of a maintenance failure occurred on board the *Canmar Spirit* (Transportation Safety Board of Canada 1999). On January 27, 1999, the container ship *Canmar Spirit* was cruising through the Port of Montreal in Canada heading toward the berthing section. As a normal part of engine duties during maneuvering, one of the engine room crew was detailed to start two of the ship's main air compressors. After starting the No. 1 compressor without incident, he proceeded to initiate the No. 3 compressor. Shortly after start-up a sudden and violent overpressurization occurred within the No. 3 compressor. The second-stage air cooler cover burst into fragments and projected outward, seriously injuring the crewmember, who later died in the hospital. The findings revealed that one of the reasons the No. 3 compressor pressure relief valves failed was due to the accumulation of sooty, oily residues. It is common practice that compressors need to undergo periodic maintenance, which is specified under the manufacturer's manual. It was evident from the findings that regular maintenance and calibration of the relief valves were not conducted. Compressors are also equipped with non-return (check) valves. Upon examination, it was found that the non-return valves on each of the three compressors were not functioning correctly. Similar to that found on the relief valves, the non-return valves were also clogged with oily, sooty residues. No documentary evidence was found to substantiate that the recommended maintenance was undertaken by the ship's crew. An operational omission (system delivery valve not opened before the compressor was started) led to the active failure. This active failure and the less than adequate maintenance, one of perhaps many latent conditions (which resulted in the malfunctioning of the air relief valves), were found to be the main contributory factors that finally aligned to result in this tragic event. This accident highlighted maintenance shortfalls in the system, which was a reflection of the overall organizational safety culture.

Most maintenance tasks share some common characteristics, which can be split into three critical steps:

1. Recognizing and understanding the maintenance tasks that are required to be performed;
2. Completing the maintenance task;
3. Checking and certifying to ensure that the maintenance task has been done correctly.

It is important that each of these steps be completed in an effective manner. Under difficult environmental conditions one or more of these critical elements may be missed, which can manifest as a latent failure. This may go undetected for a while, until the active failures combine to create an accident as happened in the case of the *Canmar Spirit*.

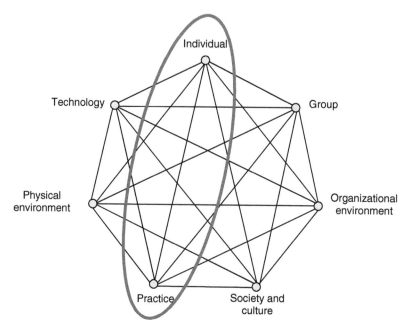

Figure 7.6 Interaction between individual and practice within the sociotechnical system model.

7.5   Practice

One important domain within the sociotechnical system model which we discuss briefly in the final section of this chapter is *practice*. As indicated in Chapter 1 and Figure 7.6, "practice" has its own distinct place in the socio-technical system model, highlighting its importance. Practice refers to such aspects as informal rules and customs and is related to the way the job is done. It is common on board that with practice crewmembers adapt to various situations and manage to solve problems they encounter on board. This can, in some circumstances, lead to an unsafe state, especially if crewmembers adopt bad practices. Hence, the importance of reviewing and updating practice and procedures periodically is crucial within the maritime domain. This is because the work on board ships is, as it is the case in other safety-critical domains, often characterized by a mismatch between procedures and practice. That is, the procedures and the way the job/task is carried out may in some cases differ.

As an example, we can mention the findings of a pilot study conducted by one of the authors in the medical domain. During the study, observations were conducted on the practice of six nurses in the handling of medicine. All six nurses had a different way of doing things (different practice). Most of them did not follow the written procedure exactly. There was one nurse, however, who did follow the procedure. This provided confirmation

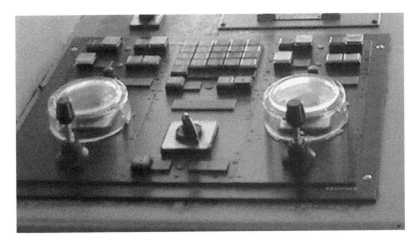

Figure 7.7 Switches covered by ashtrays to prevent use by mistake.

on the distinction that does exist between procedure and practice. Another example is based on observations by one of the authors while conducting research on a ro-ro passenger ferry. The author observed that crew did not follow the unloading procedure on the ferry. One main reason for this was time pressure. The crew wanted to perform the unloading as effectively as possible by trying to save time in order to get the vehicles back on the road as quickly as possible. The crew had developed a *practice* for efficiently unloading the ferry, but this differed from the unloading written procedure. This is not uncommon on ships, in which practice changes and adapts with experience, eventually deviating from the original written procedures. It is, however, important to note that practice is usually shaped by the procedures and checklists.

There are cases in which practice is developed from limitations of the technology identified by the crew. Figure 7.7 illustrates this using an example from a ship. The crew changed the design of a panel by gluing ashtrays from the cafeteria over switches to avoid operating them by mistake. The reason for the redesign of the panel by the crew can probably be found in their practice: once they operated the wrong switch by mistake, and it caused a dangerous situation. This led them to develop this redesign to support "better" practice.

7.6   Conclusion

It is now more important than ever that human error analysis considers the impact of organizational as well as cultural and social influences on human behavior. As highlighted in this chapter this actually entails looking beyond the direct causes of human error and focusing on the underlying organizational factors that give rise to these conditions. This chapter has described two important kinds of failure relating to human and organizational error, referred to as active and latent failures, respectively. This emphasizes the point that errors are not restricted to frontline operators of the maritime system. Cultural aspects, such as differences in national, professional, and organizational cultures, can give rise to latent failures, which may affect crew behavior and ultimately system safety. One way of inducing optimum behavior is for organizations to develop and adopt a good safety culture. An important feature of safety culture is that it is dynamic and can evolve from unsafe to safe (and sometimes vice versa). Hence, it is important that organizations keep track of their level of safety.

One crucial attribute of a good safety management system is the availability of data. To improve their safety management system and effectively strengthen defenses, organizations need data on the sources and types of errors. For example, as indicated in Chapter 1 and as explored further in Chapter 8, there is an increasing realization that a systematic analysis of minor incidents and near-miss data can yield a great amount of reliable information that can be used to improve system safety. Domains such as aviation have implemented such systems, which have been in place for years and are already providing valuable information. The maritime domain has just started implementing such reporting systems, including the Maritime Accident Investigation Branch in the United Kingdom and the U.S. Coast Guard. The collection of data entails a level of trust, which is one of the key characteristics that need to be considered, for achieving a proactive maritime safety culture. The acquisition of the necessary information allows all members of the organization (and especially management) to be proactive in improving the organization's defenses and overall system safety. Chapter 8 looks at some of the methods adopted for, and the importance of, these non-blame reporting systems.

chapter eight

Methods for data collection

8.1   Introduction

Throughout this book we have stressed the importance of collecting human factors data and operator performance information. This chapter focuses specifically on several different methods that can be used in the maritime environment to collect such data. It begins by examining some general and all-encompassing concepts, before moving on to more specific issues by examining different methods. In particular, this chapter first considers why we should collect maritime human factors data, and then it gives a general overview of methods. Following that, it goes into more detail about several data acquisition and analysis techniques. Finally, this is all tied together in a brief conclusions section.

Like many other complex sociotechnical systems, and as specified in Chapter 7, the current paradigm in maritime risk management involves developing safe systems of work, rather than looking purely at operator behavior "at the sharp end." The methods examined in this chapter therefore reflect the overall sociotechnical model used throughout this book. As seen in Chapter 1 and throughout this book, the maritime system is complex, with elements including:

- A diverse group of crew
- Commercial shipping companies from around the world
- IMO and national laws, regulations, classification standards, and guidelines
- A plethora of different maritime equipment manufacturers and suppliers
- The built environment (such as the design of ports)
- The uncertainties of the natural environment (e.g., varying currents or temperatures)

Clearly then, a wide variety of data collection methods are needed to cover the human element in all these aspects.

8.2   Why collect human factors data?

Throughout this book we have put forward the case that the application of human factors knowledge can help develop safer, more efficient, healthier, and more motivating maritime systems. To do this, however, we need to generate and apply reliable and valid human factors data. According to a classic human factors text (Sanders and McCormick 1993), human factors is largely an empirical science, applying information about people's character-istics and limitations to the design of objects, procedures, and environments. Therefore, good data collection is essential to provide the information both to develop safe and effective maritime systems, devices, and tasks and to evaluate and improve their design.

Furthermore, as we have noted throughout this book, a significant num-ber of maritime accidents* and incidents still occur, especially in develop-ing countries. Given the global nature of shipping, overall fatalities, injuries, ship losses, and equipment damage are therefore far too high. As seen in Chapter 1, human error (in its various guises) is often attributed a causal factor in a high percentage of such incidents, often around 70 to 80 percent of all occurrences. We argue that to help reduce the numbers, a greater focus on the human element in maritime operations needs to occur, and that using appropriate data gathering and analysis tools is a vital part of that focus.

Human factors data and operator performance information are not related just to accidents and incidents; other uses include the evaluation of the effectiveness of training or maritime equipment usability testing. As we have stressed throughout this book, the human element is a key aspect of maritime operations; therefore, collecting, analyzing, and applying human factors data, especially related to where "things went wrong," is vital to help develop safer, healthier, and more efficient systems of work.

8.3   An introduction to maritime human factors methods

In 1993, Sanders and McCormick broadly classified human factors studies into three types:

1. **Descriptive studies** characterize populations in terms of certain attri-butes (e.g., crew body size or engine room operator hearing loss).
2. **Experimental research** tests the effects of different variables on behav-ior (e.g., navigation officer reading speed with varying levels of myo-pia (short-sightedness).

---

* Indeed, many safety researchers do not advocate using the term "accident" as this implies some fatalistic notion that the event was somehow random, an "act of God," or just bad luck. Instead, terms like "grounding" or "contact" are being increasingly used; however, for simplicity, we will continue using the term accident in this book, with the knowledge that it does not imply a random or non-avoidable event.

3. **Evaluative research** assesses the effects of something (e.g., a new train-ing regime) on a selected criterion (e.g., crew workload or errors).

It is noted here that the investigation of accidents, incidents, near misses, and errors could perhaps be added to this list as another type of transport human factors method. Whatever the exact number of methods, such a clas-sification is useful to characterize what maritime human factors data should be collected and analyzed. As such, when deciding on collecting human fac-tors data, perhaps the most fundamental issue is to establish the purpose of the data collection. This might include examining different equipment designs (e.g., the alarms as part of an Integrated Bridge System) to choose the best one, investigating maintenance errors to learn lessons for the future, or evaluating safety procedures to design safe systems. Although exploratory studies can sometimes be useful, usually just collecting human factors data without a clear goal may lead to such data being ignored by the key decision makers in the maritime system.

8.3.1 Collecting maritime human factors data

Building on the key principles outlined by Sanders and McCormick (1993), there are other general aspects to consider when collecting maritime human factors data.

8.3.1.1 Where to conduct the study

Often this is defined by the question to be answered; however, we may need to trade off control, safety, and lower cost in a laboratory/maritime simula-tor, with the realism and motivation on board a ship. As with other areas of human factors studies, laboratory or simulator studies can offer a high level of control, whereas field studies often offer greater realism. However, we must bear in mind that in the field, data collection can often come in a poor second compared with the crew's main objective of operating the ship. Sadly, no single, perfect data collection method (or setting) exists to study maritime human factors in all its forms.

8.3.1.2 What to examine

The variables of interest could be physical, performance, subjective, or physi-ological. In experimental research they might include either task/equipment, environment (e.g., noise), or subject-related (e.g., age, sex, height) aspects. Often while examining a broad issue, composite measures may need to be obtained. For example, determining the effectiveness of new bridge resources management training might include subjective questionnaires as well as actual performance measures.

8.3.1.3   What measures to record

In human factors studies, measures are usually of three types: system descriptive (e.g., engine room equipment breakdown), task performance (e.g., quantity/quality/time to load freight), or human (performance, physiological, psychological, or subjective). Also, they can be either "terminal" (the end state, e.g., whether written warning was obeyed) or "intermediate" (e.g., if the warning was even looked at by operators).

8.3.1.4   Who to study

A sample should ideally be representative of the maritime population with the aspects we want to examine.

8.3.1.5   How to collect the data

Partly, this follows the choice of setting to collect the data (where more control is usually possible away from a working ship). Often surveys or questionnaires are used for descriptive studies, but these can have problems with low response rates by operators in maritime situations. Data collection for evaluations is often more difficult as it is often not possible to monitor or measure easily without changing the process we want to examine. The use of maritime simulators can be of great assistance here; for example, when measuring a concept referred to earlier in this book, situation awareness (SA), one approach is to interrupt the work an operator is currently doing and ask the operator to complete a questionnaire to assess his or her level of SA. As such, maritime simulators can be of great use to assess operator skills, whereas operator knowledge may be best assessed by computer-based training or instructor ratings. For reasons of practicality, some studies use random sampling. Having "enough" data in the sample depends on the degree of accuracy required, how much variability there is in the population, and how the analysis might be undertaken. Often, of course, practicalities intrude, and the sample (especially when on a ship) may be less than statistically optimal.

8.3.1.6   How to analyze the data

Some of the more common methods include descriptive studies (e.g., averages) and inferential statistics in experimental research (e.g., to assess significant differences after an intervention took place, such as training, is compared to a baseline level before the training). Later in this chapter, several analysis methods (such as human reliability analysis) will be investigated further. However, in very general terms, the focus in human factors tends to be on objective and quantitative data.

8.3.1.7   Study requirements

Ideally, human factors studies should be practical (objective, unobtrusive, easy to collect, little cost involved), reliable (consistent/stable over time/ samples), valid (measures what is intended), free from contamination by unplanned or unintended influences, and sensitive enough to answer the question posed. For example, the use of psychophysiological monitoring techniques such as galvanic skin response can be effective for quantifying the stress and strain an operator is experiencing; however, the use of such sophisticated equipment on board ships may measure factors more precisely than required, or may simply be impractical.

8.3.2   Overview of maritime human factors data collection methods

Considering the above, what data collection methods are appropriate to the maritime environment? Although not an exhaustive list, we suggest the following methods.

8.3.2.1   Accidents and incident analysis

As we examine in greater detail later, gathering and analyzing data about incidents, accidents, and near misses can be vital to help improve future safety. The Critical Incident Technique and Critical Decision Method (CDM) are knowledge elicitation techniques to analyze near misses through worker interviews and other methods. Although not formally an incident/accident collection process, in the CDM technique the aim is to uncover the processes by which a critical incident is detected and corrective action is undertaken. Such techniques may be more effective than accident investigations in developing safer systems because more of these incidents occur, so they provide more opportunities to gain insights into why problems occurred and how they can be overcome or recovered from, and workers might be more willing to talk about them (at least, if there is a "no blame" regime on board).

8.3.2.2   Simulations/human performance studies

This method more closely corresponds to the "experimental research" method mentioned above. The focus is often purely on overt responses by operators: for example, when driving vehicles in a loading area of a ship, studying the vehicle speed reductions that result from the introduction of an onboard speed restriction sign.

8.3.2.3   Eye movements/visual behavior

Again, this method falls into the experimental methods. As many maritime tasks are visual, using eye-tracking technology to record where an individual is looking when interacting with a device such as a navigation display can be valuable, say, to assess optimal layouts by means of "link analysis" (in which the sequence of glances at different display components is analyzed).

8.3.2.4   Concurrent or retrospective verbal protocols

This method involves maritime operators "thinking aloud" either during a task or while watching footage of them performing the task. This is useful to get some understanding of their decision-making processes. An example of this might be to examine expert judgment during fault diagnosis in the engine room.

8.3.2.5   *Environmental measuring*

Earlier in this book we discussed the impact of environmental variables such as noise, lighting, temperature, and vibration on operator performance and health. Measuring such parameters and comparing them to guidelines and standards can be vital in several situations, especially when a problem is suspected (e.g., bridge crew not always able to hear system alarms due to a high ambient noise level).

8.3.2.6   *Physical measuring*

Measuring key characteristics of individual operators can sometimes be vital for both new and existing ships. Such characteristics include crew body size, physical fitness, and strength. Techniques to measure physical work-load specifically are discussed in more detail later in this chapter. Other psychophysiological measures include galvanic skin responses and electro-encephalography (EEG) to more precisely quantify the amount of stress a crewmember is experiencing.

8.3.2.7   *Task analyses*

This method is undertaken to understand how tasks should officially be per-formed (and how they are actually performed by operators), the information and job aids needed for the task, and the decisions and actions required to achieve successful task completion. There are a variety of different methods, ranging from more physical descriptions of the tasks, through to those that focus on more cognitive factors. Allied to these, methods such as skill assess-ment, training needs analysis, mission analysis, predetermined time stan-dards (e.g., how long an "average" operator would take to complete a task by decomposing the task and examining how long each step in it should take), and error analysis are also becoming more formalized and commonly used.

8.3.2.8   *Checklists/standards/audits*

These are seemingly easy to administer, but often require expert judgment to apply and interpret them properly. As well as for actual operations, such techniques can also be applied to written procedures, instructions, and oper-ations manuals.

8.3.2.9   *"Walk-through" evaluations*

As the name suggests this method involves a walk-through evaluation of a product, interface, system, or procedure. This method can be combined with other methods, such as completing a checklist during the walk-through.

8.3.2.10   Computer-aided design/evaluations

This method may involve using packages such as SAMMIE® (SAMMIE CAD Limited, United Kingdom) or Jack® (UGS Corp., United States) to help model and evaluate different designs (e.g., of a new ship workstation layout) on a computer. They can allow issues such as operator reach, visibility, and control forces to be evaluated before expensive physical models are built. A lower-technology version would be to use physical mockups.

8.3.2.11   Observations

This method involves, for example, observing the number and type of verbal communications between operators in the engine room or investigating usability defects with a new item of equipment. Depending on the situation, observations can be continuous or sampled (often when critical events are likely, e.g., during emergency drills). Observations can be usefully supplemented with video/static images, sound recordings, or checklists/recording sheets, but such recordings should not interfere with the issue under investigation.

8.3.2.12   Interviews/focus groups/questionnaires

This method, which entails talking to people and asking questions, is perhaps the most obvious method available. For example, these tools may be used to assess the attitudes of a group to a particular safety issue, such as safety climate on a ship. Interviews have varying degrees of structure depending on their purpose (e.g., they may be less structured and have more open questions when an investigator wishes to get an overview of a topic). All these techniques are seemingly intuitive; however, unless great care is taken to decide the purpose, format (often including pilot testing), and analysis method in advance, they can be expensive and inefficient. As will be seen later in this chapter, questionnaires can also be useful for investigating issues such as crew mental workload.

8.3.2.13   Log books

Often log books can be thought of as a longer-term questionnaire that is self-administered. Depending on the study, they may be completed by the crew hourly, daily, or weekly, to investigate issues such as longer-term trends in fatigue levels, training success, or opinions and views of ship habitability.

8.4   Application of data acquisition and analysis techniques to key human factors issues

Based on the above overview of the types of maritime human factors data collection methods available, this section reviews in more depth techniques that can be applied to several key issues that have been highlighted earlier in the book.

8.4.1   Fatigue

As we previously noted, operator fatigue can be a major factor on ships. However, unlike other temporary impairments such as alcohol (which can be measured by the blood alcohol content as indicated in Chapter 3), there is no direct way of measuring fatigue. We can only measure the "indicators" of fatigue, not fatigue itself. Indicators that might be suitable for maritime data collection include:

- Quantity of work, for example, amount of freight checked by a maritime operator in an hour
- Quality of work, such as the types, timing, and severity of errors made
- Subjective reports, for example, asking operator if they are fatigued by means of interview, questionnaire, or log book
- Specialized physiological monitoring devices, for example, "brainwaves," EEGs, or visual measures
- Specialized psychological tasks, for example, on-screen tracking or reaction time tasks

Operator fatigue detection and prediction technologies (e.g., devices that estimate or predict fatigue based on either the maritime operator's state or behavior) are currently areas of significant research and development work. However, as yet, most devices are still not sufficiently evaluated for them to be used extensively in maritime operations.

8.4.2   Workload

Earlier in this book we saw how workload (both mental and physical) is a key factor influencing human performance in the maritime environment. As such, several methods to measure both types of workload are briefly considered below.

8.4.2.1   Physical workload

Heavy work is characterized by high energy consumption and severe stresses on the heart and lungs. The limits to performance of heavy work are largely set by an operator's energy consumption and cardiac capacity as described in Chapter 3, and these two functions are often used to assess the severity of a physical task.

Basal metabolism is the consumption of energy a person uses when lying down with an empty stomach. For a 70-kilogram man this amounts to about 7,000 kilojoules (kJ) per 24 hours. As physical work increases, then so does energy demand. Increased energy consumption in a task can be expressed in work joules, and determined by measuring energy consumption while working and subtracting basal metabolism. For example, a physical task like manually loading on board a ship may use 18,500 kJ per shift, so subtracting the basal level of 7,000 kJ gives work joules as 11,500 kJ. This process, of course, tells us only about energy use for strenuous physical work, so should not be used for studying mental activities or detailed skilled work. Energy consumption of 20,000 kJ per working day (averaged over a long period of several months) can be considered to be a reasonable maximum, although this can vary with factors such as age, constitution, and seasonal workload on the ship.

Heart rate is another measure of physical workload, with a rise in heart rate related to energy consumption for a given task. Measuring heart rate is one of the most useful ways of assessing physical workload, because it can be done so easily (as compared with many other psychophysiological measures), for example, by operators wearing a simple sensor around their chest. However, the rise in heart rate with increasing workload is greater when the ambient temperature is higher, so ambient temperature should also be recorded to obtain an accurate measure of workload.

8.4.2.2 Mental workload

By assessing the levels of mental workload required by various maritime tasks, it is possible to arrange, schedule, or even alter tasks in such a way that performance can be optimized. Mental workload assessment methods include:

- Primary task measures: Direct observation (e.g., timing of maritime task performance).
- Secondary task measures: A second (e.g., memory) task is performed simultaneously, and its effect on performance of the primary task (or both tasks) is studied.
- Comparative measures: When, for example, introducing a new device on a ship, workload data from a predecessor system can be used to compare against data for the new system.
- Simulation models: Mathematical models using human performance data can provide workload estimates, although the accuracy of the model used is critical.
- Psychophysiological measures (e.g., eye-blink reflexes): These can be useful, but as mentioned earlier, these often require a lot of equipment or a laboratory setting.
- Subjective measures: Ask the operator (e.g., questionnaires with rating scales about mental effort, stress, and timing). Examples include the Subjective Workload Assessment Technique (SWAT) and NASA Task Load Index (NASA-TLX). As a note of caution, these may be influenced by factors such as bias or opinions of the operator.
- Task analysis methods: Decomposition of overall system goals into segments, operator tasks, and task requirements. One commonly used method in the military domain is a time-based breakdown of demands on the maritime operator (that is, the amount of mental resources required per unit time relative to those available). Hierarchical task

analysis (HTA), goals, operators, methods, and selection rules (GOMS), and cognitive task analysis are other examples of task analytic methods; however, further consideration of them is outside the scope of this book. Likewise, more advanced analysis methods, such as cognitive work analysis, are becoming increasingly popular in academic and professional maritime research institutes; however, the training required to master such methods, as well as the time required to perform such analyses, puts them beyond the reach of many practitioners.

8.4.3 Accident analysis and the importance of incident and near-miss data

Maritime incident/accident investigation is usually a complex process that needs to be undertaken by skilled professionals, ideally with some human factors training. For example, in Australia, this includes professionals from the Australian Transport Safety Bureau and the Defence Science and Technology Organisation, with similar bodies in Europe, the United States, and elsewhere. Part of the complexity lies in the nature of the accident; there are often many causal factors and error antecedents. Collecting accident data and conducting appropriate analyses require specialized skills and experience, as well as a large number of resources. Data collection methods include obtaining data from systems recorders (e.g., voice recorders on bridges), written documents (e.g., training documents, audits, certificates, and standard operating procedures), and interviews with all those involved in different aspects of the ship system, such as crew, supervisors, ship managers and operators, flag state, classification society, regulators, and designers. Further, accident data are only as good as the collection tools used to obtain the data.

When data have been collected, a large number of accident investigation and error analysis techniques exist; two that we discuss later in this chapter are the management oversight risk tree (MORT) and human reliability assessment (HRA). Other techniques include barrier analysis, fault tree analysis, and timeline analysis. Some techniques focus on active and latent factors, others on failures of human information processing, and others on contributing factors. As can perhaps be gathered from this, sadly, in maritime accident investigation there is still no widespread agreement on concepts or methods and techniques, although the sociotechnical model used in this book could be a useful framework to promote such agreement. However, the conclusions about what happened, why it happened, what should be done about it in the future, and how those recommendations are put into action should be similar irrespective of the exact analysis technique used.

Accident investigation is often mandated by international agreements or may be required for insurance or certification purposes, but for all concerned the main philosophy behind it should be to learn lessons from these past incidents. The results of these investigations should be used to implement effective risk reduction strategies to help guard against future negative events (or at least to mitigate their severity). As we know, human error is cited as a cause of a large number of maritime incidents and accidents; as such, investigations need to take into account what is known on the origins of, and antecedents to, both human and organizational error. Over recent years a growing body of documents, guidelines, and resolutions has become available to assist an investigator to focus on the human element in shipping accidents. These include some classification societies (such as the American Bureau of Shipping, or ABS), European Commission-sponsored projects, and the International Maritime Organization (IMO). For example, the IMO (2000) Resolution.A884 (21) amends the code for the investigation of marine casualties and incidents to focus more on the investigation of human factors. These guidelines provide a systematic approach to considering the human element, based on established human error frameworks. The general process is in six steps (IMO 2000):

1. **Collect data of the occurrence.** It is especially important to use a systematic approach to ensure that critical information is not lost or overlooked. As such, this stage focuses on "what, who, and when?" type questions.
2. **Determine the sequence of the occurrence.** Organizing the data collected in step 1 to re-create the sequence of events and circumstances. As such the process is now focused on more latent/background "how and why?" type questions.
3. **Identify unsafe conditions and unsafe acts or decisions.** The above information is used to discover causal factors in the occurrence.

Then for each unsafe act or decision the process delves deeper:

4. **Identify the type of error or violation.** For example, this may specify the act was due to an intended violation as opposed to an unintended slip.
5. **Identify the underlying factors.** It is important to note that for each act or decision there may often be more than one underlying factor.
6. **Identify potential safety issues and develop appropriate safety actions.** Based on all the above, the final stage is to identify the safety issues involved, and (perhaps most importantly) propose safety actions.

Overall, Resolution.A884 (21) provides a reasonable amount of valuable human factors support to the investigator. For example, it suggests types of human factors questions that may help the investigator; these include questions about crew training, operator duties, level of ship automation, workload, and work–rest cycles (in fact, many of the issues covered in this book).

8.4.3.1 Maritime accident reports

At present masters and/or ship operators are required to report serious accidents (usually classified as very serious casualties or serious casualties) to their respective maritime authorities; less serious events are encouraged to be submitted where important lessons may be learned. In some countries, a procedure for reporting incidents and near misses has also been developed, but this is currently conducted on a voluntary basis. Over the past ten years or so, the IMO and other bodies have further standardized the reporting and investigation procedures, and have placed a stronger emphasis on human factors issues like individual errors and fatigue in their different reporting forms. Also, it should be noted that the findings from maritime accident reports are sometimes used to consider new legislation and procedures by the IMO in order to enhance maritime safety; indeed, the accident forms often encourage comment about how the findings of an accident investigation may affect international regulations. Finally, some of the major maritime administrations openly publish accident reports on their Web sites, which are available for download by the public. All this is encouraging: the accident data collection and analyses processes are improving and a more specific emphasis on human factors is emerging. However, as will be seen below, there is plenty of work yet to be done in this area.

Some authorities publishing maritime accident/incident reports in English are:

- Marine Accident Investigation Branch (www.maib.gov.uk)
- Transportation Safety Board of Canada (www.tsb.gc.ca)
- Transportation Accident Investigation Commission (www.taic.org.nz)
- Swedish Accident Investigation Board (www.havkom.se)
- Danish Maritime Authority, The Division for Investigation of Maritime Accidents (www.dma.dk)
- National Transportation Safety Board (www.ntsb.gov)
- Maritime New Zealand (www.msa.govt.nz)
- Australian Transport Safety Bureau (www.atsb.gov.au)
- The Nautical Institute Marine Accident Reporting Scheme MARS (www.nautinst.org/MARS/)
- U.S. Coast Guard Casualty Reports (www.uscg.mil/hq/g-m/)

8.4.3.2 Accident versus incident and near-miss data

There is a need in the maritime domain to recognize the inevitability of individual errors by operators; however, the prevailing safety culture is such that this fact is sometimes still not recognized in the design, construction, and operations of ships. Attempting to eliminate future errors by just looking at the underlying causes of similar errors is a very difficult task. As mentioned above, analysis of accident reports is one way to attempt to do so. Although the area is evolving fast, the use of maritime accident (or casualty) data can still be problematic for several reasons. First, casualties are rare events and hence only limited information can be retrieved from these, apart from the fact that analysis of these accident reports can be a very time-consuming task. Second, despite having some common aspects, maritime casualty investigation practices still differ across countries in terms of the precise methods and procedures utilized (including how the data are subsequently coded, stored, and retrieved), making comparisons problematic. Third, information contained in maritime accident reports is not always consistent or detailed enough; this is demonstrated by an occasional lack of focus on organizational error aspects. Individual errors are becoming better catered to, but may still not contain sufficient detail to directly inform future system countermeasures on ships, or more general maritime safety policy measures. Finally, investigators may be experts in a specific maritime technical area, but they often have minimal knowledge (formal or otherwise) of human factors in accident causation and safety management.

One way of partly reducing some of these distorting effects is to study incidents or near misses. As mentioned earlier, the CDM is one way of examining near misses and crew system difficulties. It is designed to collect data in naturalistic settings and focuses on critical events. Since inception, this technique has undergone a number of modifications and has been used in such studies as aircraft equipment operations, long-haul truck operations, and nuclear power plant control room operations. Taking into account that CDM has been used in a variety of domains it is now generally viewed as a well-validated technique; however, up until now there has been fairly limited use of this technique in the maritime domain.

Another approach is to examine incident and near-miss reports (where they exist), independent from accident (casualty) reports. This can provide more insight, because as described in Chapter 1 the number of near misses and incidents is naturally much larger than that of accidents. However, data can be limited. At present, such a system is a long way from realization in many maritime operations, so to gather such data means an independent near-miss reporting and analysis system needs to be set up, and the safety culture of a ship and the ship owner and/or operator needs to be such that near misses are openly reported.

To conclude, the study of accident, incidents, and near misses is a key method (or series of methods) to collect and analyze maritime human factors data. Despite progress over the past ten years, the data available are still far from perfect. Of course, to some degree such a criticism could be leveled at other domains such as aviation or rail safety; however, the maritime industry still lags behind these fields in many regards. Part of the problem is that, as mentioned in Chapter 7, the dominant maritime culture is still concerned with compliance and blame assignment, rather than independent and objective fact-finding to improve future operations and policy.

8.4.4 Human reliability analysis

HRA is closely related to the above discussion about accidents and near misses. As an overall methodology, HRA is a procedure for conducting a quantitative analysis to predict operator error. As a measure, it is the probability of successful performance of a task or element of a task (often expressed as a probability figure, e.g., 0.992). HRA began in the 1950s when there was a desire to quantify the human element in a system. Since then, many attempts have been made to develop databases of human reliability information (especially in the nuclear and other high-hazard industries).

There are several specific methodologies to determine human reliability. Like accident analysis, there is no single, commonly accepted approach. For example, the Technique for Human Error Rate Prediction (THERP) breaks down a task into sub-steps, and then provides probabilities for successful task performance from databases, which are then combined with expert judgments to determine the human reliability for the whole system being analyzed. Computer systems exist where a task or series of tasks can be simulated—so it is possible to run the simulation to see the effects of making a change; for example, would more errors occur if time to complete a task was reduced.

MORT is another risk analysis methodology that can have a significant human factors component. The analysis is undertaken by means of a fault tree, where the top event is the accident/critical event under investigation. The tree arrangement gives an indication of the causes of the top event from oversights and omissions by management and/or from assumed risks. In the maritime field, MORT can be primarily used in the analysis or investigation of accidents and incidents, although it can also be used in the evaluation of safety programs. MORT can be highly effective in identifying underlying management root causes of hazards; however, it can be time consuming and costly to use.

A full review of such techniques is outside the scope of this book. However, some of the problems with HRA and related techniques (especially the more quantitative techniques) are that people are variable and therefore the obtained numbers may be of limited value in some cases, that not all errors result in failure (recovery is possible), that the specific HRA methodologies are not always well validated, that it is not possible to verify to the level of precision claimed (e.g., 0.992), that many techniques still rely on subjective/expert judgment to give weights, and that not enough maritime human performance data exist for their widespread use. However, although not perfect, HRA techniques are sometimes useful to give overall working estimates of either current or prospective ship systems, or to systematically evaluate the specific control, individual, and management factors that caused or contributed to a maritime accident. Therefore, it is hoped that more work to develop, evaluate, and apply such methods will continue.

8.4.5   Safety climate/safety culture questionnaires and surveys

As we saw in Chapter 7, the notion of safety culture covers a wide range of characteristics that include personnel attitudes and the control, management, and organization of maritime work activities. Although different maritime companies have different organizational structures, the important characteristics of safety culture include members of the company having an open and questioning attitude, all staff having shared perceptions of the importance of safety, using effective training, having personal accountability, demonstrating adherence to procedures, using systematic management processes, and having the willingness to learn from past experience. Different shipping companies have different organizational cultures; however, the linkage between poor maritime safety culture and increased accident liability is now generally well accepted.

There are a variety of quantitative and qualitative tools available to measure safety culture; these include safety climate questionnaires, observing work safety behaviors, and using safety audits. Perhaps the most commonly used method is by questionnaire; in the maritime field these include the appropriately named Maritime Culture Questionnaire and the Maritime Climate Questionnaire. Although maritime safety culture is vitally important, and can be reasonably easily measured, it can be very difficult to change. Both management and operator resistance to change, peer pressure, perception of the apparent costs of change, and a lack of understanding of safety risks are all likely to be factors against change.

8.5   *Cost–benefit analysis and human factors*

We end this chapter by outlining a broad approach to consider the costs and benefits of human factors initiatives. Historically, human factors/ergonomics arose out of military applications, where justifying the exact economic costs of human factors work, compared to its likely benefits, was often not a high priority. The maritime industry today is, however, very concerned about costs, and many organizations work on very small profit margins. Hence, many human factors interventions need to be justified in terms of their likely benefits exceeding their anticipated costs. Cost–benefit analysis is an area where ergonomists and human factors specialists have not traditionally been very strong; this applies as much to the maritime industry as it does to other domains. But in the current economic climate it is vital to compare the money spent on human factors work with the benefits such work produces.

Human factors interventions in most industries (of course, including the maritime one) usually have the dual objectives of increasing productivity/effectiveness and improving the conditions of work (for operator safety, health, comfort, and convenience). Although consideration may be given to ease of use, comfort, and the like, most of the analysis is done on both short- to medium-term performance and safety benefits. Such an approach does not usually fully consider long-term environmental costs (e.g., from the spillage of cargo due to a human error).

Ideally, the measures of effectiveness (i.e., performance and safety aspects) would be gathered both before and after the intervention was implemented; thus a comparison could be made to assess how successful the intervention was, and this could be compared to the intervention cost. However, examining the topic in more detail shows that undertaking maritime human factors cost–benefit analysis is often problematic; some of these difficulties are (adapted from Rouse and Boff 1997):

- Investments or costs of maritime human factors interventions often occur long before returns are realized. Thus benefits are delayed, obscured by time, or are no longer relevant.
- Benefits are seldom purely monetary (e.g., ease of use of a new device on the bridge, or improved operator working conditions).
- Costs and benefits are often distributed among a wide range of stakeholders (e.g., for a new device on the bridge, this may include the operators, supervisors, maintenance workers, ship managers, and company accountants). Thus, input from all of these groups is necessary.
- Benefits might be related to events that do not happen, such as ship accidents being avoided due to good human factors design. If the same type of intervention were implemented on many ships, then a reduced trend in the accident rate may be discernible; however, this would require both a large number of ships and a long period of data collection.
- Most ships are complex systems, so the effect of improvements to one small part of the system (e.g., better engine room controls and displays) might be methodologically difficult to assess.

Rouse and Boff (1997) argue that a structured method to assess the cost–benefits of human factors is needed. As part of this, they argue that it is necessary to define the types of human factors benefits more exactly. They state that these benefits can range from the very tangible to the less tangible, so in the case of maritime operations this may include:

Most Tangible
- Solution not otherwise possible (e.g., a ship incapable of operation)
- Acceptable performance/cost not otherwise possible (such as a ship unable to safely cruise at higher speeds)
- Improved operator performance and/or cost savings (e.g., reduced fuel use)
- Enhanced customer willingness to pay (e.g., for freight on container vessels)
- Cost/mishaps avoidance (e.g., fewer errors during routine maintenance)
- Increased confidence by all those involved in the maritime system
Least Tangible

Thus, there are substantial difficulties associated with cost–benefit assessment of maritime human factors work. Applying a structured methodology that emphasizes what should be represented in the analysis can improve the situation. Despite this, obtaining quantitative figures is either impossible or at best imprecise. But such figures (albeit imperfect) can at least be useful in comparing between alternative strategies. To summarize:

> it is always worthwhile to think in terms of costs and benefits. It is always useful to think about stakeholders and the attributes that concern them. It is always valuable to think about who benefits, how these benefits will get to them, and what these benefits will be worth. It is better yet when these questions can be answered quantitatively. (Rouse and Boff 1997, p. 1632)

It is hoped that as the maritime human factors subject grows, more systematic and persuasive cost–benefit analyses will emerge.

8.6   Conclusions

This chapter has covered a wide range of material. It should be clear that which method is the most suitable for collecting and analyzing maritime human factors data depends on why the information needs to be collected, and how it will be used. As a ship is a complex system, the selection and employment of appropriate data collection methods are often far from straightforward. It is hoped that consideration of the material presented in this chapter will aid the process of collecting and analyzing reliable and valid maritime human factors data.

chapter nine

The future:
Trends in maritime human factors

Human factors knowledge and skills started to be properly introduced into the maritime domain in the 1990s. The inspiration for this was mainly due to the successful introduction of human factors training in aviation in the 1980s. As indicated in Chapter 7, the introduction of human factors was primarily focused around crew resource management (CRM) and bridge team management (BTM) training. This was also considered important in relation to investigation of maritime accidents and incidents. Such training, however, largely focused on the individual, and as highlighted in Chapter 1, human error was a frequently used term. The assumption was that it was possible to prevent human error and thereby improve safety through human factors and psychology training, using CRM and BRM courses. In many cases this was true: human factors training programs worked, bridge discipline was improved, and awareness about human capabilities and limitations was increased.

There was a tendency to focus on specific human factors issues, for example, fatigue, in which particular interest was given to this by the International Maritime Organization (IMO). Indeed, for the purposes of obtaining funding to conduct maritime interventions, or using the domain knowledge of the individual researchers, this approach was attractive. Concepts like situation awareness have also been used in attempts to find a universal explanation of human error and accidents, and communication has in some contexts been denominated the most important human factors issue. Of course, the problem with this approach was that by focusing on one issue, such as fatigue, situation awareness, or communication, masked other relevant problems.

Fortunately, in the last decade, the focus has changed from an individual perspective to a systems perspective. The organizational accident causation model formulated by James Reason in 1997 contributed to this change of perspective. As indicated by Reason (1997) it was important to look at the underlying factors in the organization acting as the basis for the human factors problems. Insufficient supervision, poor procedures, and organizational pressures were mentioned as important factors; these were highlighted in Chapter 7.

The systems perspective also includes an interest for the design of technology and equipment. Was it easy and fail-safe to use? The problem was that maritime equipment, unlike consumer products, was designed for highly technical people to use in a professional context (such as on the bridge or engine control room). The development of user-friendly products had therefore, wrongly, been seen as a non-issue in this industry. The interest for better design of equipment was primarily limited to research projects, to projects funded by the European Union and similar groups (such as the U.S. Coast Guard), and to special working groups.

Traditional CRM and BRM courses focused mostly on training of skills and transfer of knowledge of onboard crew. The underlying assumption was that crew behavior can be changed through training and acquisition of knowledge, which included an increased awareness about human factors. This was true to a certain extent. But then another concept was introduced: the concept of safety culture, referred to in Chapter 7. This changed the focus, in the sense that behavior can be changed through a change in attitudes, and "thinking safety" should hence be integrated throughout the whole organization. Thus, to facilitate the creation of a good safety culture, managers and on-shore staff were also being included in CRM and BRM training courses. Systems for the collection of data about near misses, accidents, and incidents were established as part of these programs, with the aim of improving safety culture.

The basis for the new paradigm in human factors intervention was set. From training and educating the individual to system-wide intervention programs including involvement at different organizational levels, improvement of safety culture, establishment of systems for collecting and analyzing data on near misses, accidents and incidents, training and education of management and on-shore staff, improvement of procedures and organization of work, and so forth. These programs were driven by the shipping companies as they realized the advantages gained from a human factors integration approach within the whole organization.

Improvements in equipment and technology were not normally a part of these programs, but the interest in integrating human factors knowledge among developers and manufacturers of maritime equipment increased. It was now not a matter of cumbersome manuals for the equipment, and training the crew in their use. The benefits from better user interfaces became clear, even to the manufacturers of the equipment. This led to a more formal introduction of human factors knowledge and test methods in the development process of maritime equipment.

Figures 9.1, 9.2, 9.3, and 9.4 illustrate how a simple so-called mockup made of cardboard was used in a maritime simulator to test the usability of a maritime very high frequency (VHF) radio. In the test the captain pretended to use the VHF as a real piece of equipment and made verbal reflections (thinking aloud) about the problems he encountered. The designer and human factors experts worked together observing the experiments, taking notes for improving the design.

It is likely that such usability experiments with user interfaces will gain further interest among manufacturers of maritime equipment. The result will inevitably be better, more intuitive, and more fail-safe user interfaces.

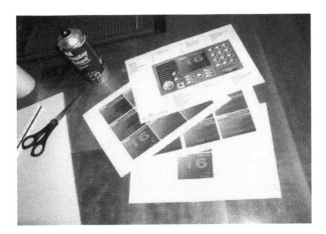

Figure 9.1 Mockup cardboard cutouts for usability test of VHF radio.

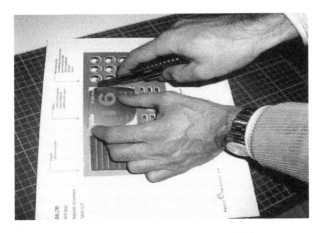

Figure 9.2 Mockup cardboard VHF radio being assembled.

New functions, improving the ease of use and accounting for specific human factors capabilities, will be introduced. For example, the experiments with the VHF mentioned above showed that the user could benefit from a built-in "memory"—a replay function—in the VHF. This would make it possible for the user to replay important messages if information was lost during the first transmission of the message (a very common problem in the use of VHF). This function is now a built-in feature of the VHF, and crewmembers around the world using VHF will appreciate the possibility of being able to hear a message again without having to ask the sender to repeat it.

Maritime human factors systems and processes are being developed largely on the basis of similar practices in aviation, defense, and nuclear power plants. Human factors knowledge and skills are now employed in

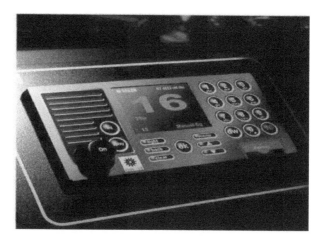

Figure 9.3   Mockup cardboard VHF Radio fitted in a maritime simulator.

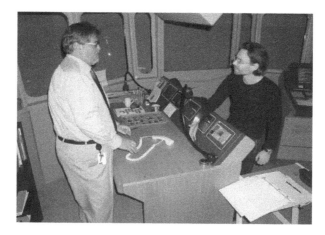

Figure 9.4   Mockup cardboard VHF radio used in a maritime simulator for usability testing.

many safety-critical domains including railways, road transport, oil and gas production, and hospitals. This dissemination of human factors knowledge will cross-fertilize in the maritime domain, contributing to new results, more sophisticated data collection and analysis methods, and innovative discoveries. This is possible because many human factors problems are of a general nature and not related to a specific domain. For example, introducing new technology into an existing work process often changes the nature of the task and modifies the role of the operator from directly acting on the system to passively monitoring it. Human factors issues in one domain will therefore often be relevant in other domains as well. And when human factors know-how is applied in many domains, the results can benefit all domains.

It is hard to say with certainty what the future in maritime human factors holds. The systems perspective and human factors intervention programs are already important trends, together with an extended focus on usability and user-centered design in the development of maritime equipment. Increases in automation and technological complexity in shipping will be further ammunition for the continued integration of human factors knowledge in the design of maritime technology. But we should still keep in mind that differences in technological complexity and automation level within the maritime domain can vary widely. For example, state-of-the-art American cruise liners with all the latest technology differ greatly from thirty- or forty-year-old cargo vessels operating in the developing world. Human factors will therefore have different priorities in different parts of the world. The discipline will probably spread and gain priority, but the research, development, and application of human factors knowledge will continue at different rates around the world with the more developed countries (such as Europe, the United States, Japan, Australia, etc.) leading the way.

References

Anderson, P. 2002. *Managing Safety at Sea*. PhD Thesis. Middlesex University: UK.

Bainbridge, L. 1987. Ironies of automation. In *New technology and human error*, ed. J. Rasmussen, K. Duncan, and J. Leplat. Chichester: Wiley (reprint of a 1983 *Automatica* paper).

Berne, E. 1961. *Transactional analysis in psychotherapy: A systematic individual and social psychiatry*. London: Evergreen Books.

Berne, E. 1964. *Games people play. The basic handbook of Transactional Analysis*. New York: Ballantine books.

BERTRANC Project. 2000. *Final consolidated progress report*. Brussels: EC.

Cantwell, V. 1997. *Physiological factors affecting safety in maritime operations*. Paper presented at Safety at Sea International '97 Conference (SASMEX), Baltimore, MD, 30 Apr to 1 May 1997.

Colquhoun, W. P., Blake, M. J., and Edwards, R. S. 1969. *Experimental studies of watchkeeping: Summary report* (Summary Report No. OES 513). Cambridge: Royal Naval Personnel Research Committee.

Dekker, S. 2002. *The field guide to human error investigations*. Aldershot, UK: Ashgate.

Dekker, S. 2005. *Ten questions about human error. A new view of human factors and system safety*. Mahwah, NJ: Lawrence Erlbaum Associates.

Dekker, S. W. A. 2000. Crew situation awareness in high-tech settings: Tactics for research into an ill-defined phenomenon. *Transportation Human Factors* 2(1): 49–62.

Edwards, E. 1972. Man and machine: Systems for safety. In *Proceedings of British Airline Pilots Associations Technical Symposium*, 21–36. London: British Airline Pilots Associations.

Endsley, M. R. 2002. Theoretical underpinnings of situation awareness: A critical review. In *Situation awareness analysis and measurement*, ed. M. R. Endsley and D. J. Garland, 3–32. Mahwah, NJ: Lawrence Erlbaum Associates.

Endsley, M. R., Bolte, B., and Jones D. G. 2003. *Designing for situation awareness*. London: Taylor & Francis.

European Commission. 1998. *Man/Ship Interface System II* (MASIS) (Final Report): Brussels: EC.

Fisch, B. J. 1999. *Fisch & Spehlmann's EEG Primer*. 3rd rev. ed. Amsterdam: Elsevier.

Flin, R. 2005. *Safe in their hands? Licensing and competence assurance for safety-critical roles in high risk industries*. Industrial Psychology Research Centre University of Aberdeen, http://www.abdn.ac.uk/iprc/papers%20reports/Safe_In_Their_Hands_Revalidation_ Report.pdf.

Furnham, A. 1997. *The psychology of behaviour at work. The individual in the organization*. Hove, UK Taylor & Francis.

Gomes, C. R., De Brito, C., Boxer, R., and Blackmore, J. 2001. (Eds) *The tragic history of the sea, 1589–1622*, trans. C. R. Boxer. University of Minnesota Press.

Grandjean, E. 1998. *Fitting the task to the man: A textbook of occupational ergonomics*, US Taylor & Francis. 4th Edition.

Grech, M. R., Horberry, T., and Smith, A. 2002. *Human error in maritime operations: Analyses of accident reports using the Leximancer tool*. Paper presented at the 46th Annual Meeting of the Human Factors and Ergonomics Society, Baltimore, MD.

Grech, M. R. 2004. *Human error in maritime operations: Assessment of situation awareness, fatigue, workload and stress*. PhD diss., University of Queensland.

Hardwick, C. 2000. *A comparative assessment of priorities for accommodation standards between Royal Naval and Merchant Naval fleets*. Paper presented at the Human Factors in Ship Design and Operations, London.

Hawkins, F. H. 1987. *Human factors in flight*. Aldershot, UK: Gower Technical Press.

Helmreich, R. L., and Merritt, A. C. 2004. *Culture at work in aviation and medicine*. Hants, UK: Ashgate.

Hofstede, G. 1980. *Culture's consequences: International differences in work-related values*. Beverly Hills, CA: Sage.

Hofstede, G. 1997. *Cultures and organisations, software of the mind—Intercultural co-operation and its importance for survival*. London: McGraw-Hill.

Hofstede, G. 2001. *Culture's consequences: Comparing values, behaviors, institutions and organizations across nations*. Thousand Oaks, CA: Sage.

Hudson, P. 2001. Safety culture: The ultimate goal. *Flight Safety Australia* Sept–Oct: 2–31.

ICAO. 2006. ECCAIRS 4.2.6 service pack 1 data definition standard. Explanatory factors, Jan 4, 2007. In *ADREP 2000 taxonomy*, International Civil Aviation Organisation (ICAO) and Joint Research Centre (JRC), http://eccairs-www.jrc.it/ICAO/ADREP2000-English/R4CDExplanatoryFactors.pdf.

International Ergonomics Association. 2007. Retrieved 15 Jan, http://www.iea.cc/.

International Maritime Organization. 1982. Resolution A.468(XII), *Code on noise levels on board ship*. London: IMO.

International Maritime Organization. 1993. Resolution A.752(18), *Guidelines for the evaluation, testing and application of low-location lighting on passenger ships*. London: IMO.

International Maritime Organization. 2000. Resolution A.884(21). *Amendments to the code for the investigation of marine casualties and incidents*. London: IMO.

International Maritime Organization. 2001. MSC/Circ. 1014, *Guidance on Fatigue Mitigation and Management*. London: 1MO.

International Maritime Organization. 2003. MSC 77/17, *Role of the human element. Definition of Safety Culture*. Submited by the UK. London: IMO.

International Standards Organization. 1996. International Standard 2923: *Acoustics—Measurement of noise on board vessels*. Geneva: ISO.

International Standards Organization. 2000. International Standard 6954: *Mechanical vibration—Guidelines for the measurement, reporting and evaluation of vibration with regard to habitability on passenger and merchant ships*. Geneva: ISO.

Klein, G. A. 1998. *Sources of power: How people make decisions*. Cambridge, MA: MIT Press.

Kleitman, N., and Jackson, P. D. 1950. *Variations in body temperature and in performance under different watch schedules* (Report NM 004005.01.02). Bethesda, MD: Naval Medical Research Institute.

Knudsen, F. 1985. *Samtalen og dens forståelsesproblemer: Voksenpædagogiske forelæsninger*. [*The discourse and its comprehensibility problems: Lectures about the teaching of adults*]. Copenhagen: Danish University of Education.

Koester, T. 2003. Situation awareness and situation dependent behaviour adjustment in the maritime work domain. In *Human-centred computing. Cognitive, social and ergonomic aspects*, vol 3, 255–9. *Proceedings of HCI-International*, Crete, Greece, 22–27 June.

Koester, T. 2007. *Terminology work in maritime human factors. Situations and socio-technical systems*. Copenhagen: Frydenlund Publishers.

Kroemer, K. H. E., and Grandjean, E. 1997. *Fitting the task to the human.* 5th ed. London: Taylor & Francis.

Lawther, A., and Griffin, M. J. 1988. Motion sickness and motion characteristics of vessels at sea. *Ergonomics* 31(10): 1373–94.

Lloyd's Register Fairplay 2004. *Total ship losses by numbers,* www.marisec.org/shippingfacts/safety/ship_losses.php.

Mara, T. D. 1969. Marine collision avoidance: Human factors considerations for the development and operation of an effective merchant marine radar. *Navigation: Journal of the Institute of Navigation* 16(1): 21–28.

Marine Accident Investigation Branch. 2001a. *Bridge watchkeeping safety study.* London: Marine Accident Investigation Branch.

Marine Accident Investigation Branch. 2001b. Report name: *P&OSL Aquitaine* (27/2001). Downloaded 27 Mar 2007, http://www.maib.gov.uk/publications/investigation_reports/2001/p_osl_aquataine.cfm.

Maritime Transportation Research Board. 1976. *Human error in merchant marine safety* (Report). Washington, DC: National Academy of Sciences.

Marshall, G. 2006. *Governance & safety management.* Paper presented at the Swinburne University Multimodal Symposium on Safety Management and Human Factors, Melbourne.

Metze, E., and Nystrup, J. 1984. *Samtaletræning: Håndbog i præcis kommunikation [Discourse training: Handbook in precise communication].* Copenhagen: Munksgaard.

Panel on Psychology and Physiology. 1949. *A survey report on human factors in undersea warfare.* Washington, DC: Committee on Undersea Warfare National Research Council.

Potter, J. O. 1992. *The* Sultana *tragedy: America's greatest maritime disaster.* 2nd ed. Gretna, LA: Pelican.

Pyne, R., and Koester, T. 2005. Methods and means for analysis of crew communication in the maritime domain. *The Archives of Transport* 17(3–4): 193–208.

Rasmussen, J. 1981. *Human errors. A taxonomy for describing human malfunction in industrial installations.* Roskilde: Risø National Laboratory, Denmark.

Reason, J. 1997. *Managing the risks of organisational accidents.* New York: Ashgate.

Riordan, C. A., Johnson, G. D., and Thomas, J. S. 1991. Personality and stress at sea. *Journal of Social Behaviour and Personality* 6(7): 391–409.

Rizzo, A., and Save, L. 1999. SHELFS: A proactive method for managing safety issues. Paper presented at RTO HFM Workshop on *"The human factor in system reliability—Is human performance predictable?"* Siena, Italy, 1–2 Dec. Published in RTO MP-032.

Rouse, W. B., and Boff, K. R. 1997. Assessing cost/benefit of human factors. In *Handbook of human factors and ergonomics,* ed. G. Salvendy. 2nd ed. New York: John Wiley.

Rowley, I., Williams, R., Barnett, M., Pekcan, C., Gatfield, D. Northcott, L., and Crick, J. 2006. *MCA RP545: Development of guidance for the mitigation of human error in automated ship-borne maritime systems.* Unclassified report QinetiQ, UK.

Sanders, M. S., and McCormick, E. J. 1993. *Human factors in engineering and design.* 7th ed. New York: McGraw-Hill.

Sarter, N. B., and Woods, D. D. 1991. Situation awareness: A critical but ill-defined phenomenon. *International Journal of Aviation Psychology* 1(1): 45–57.

Shappell, S. A., and Wiegmann, D. A. 2000. *The human factors analysis and classification system (HFACS)* (Final report DPT/FAA/AM-00/7). Oklahoma City, OK: University of Illinois at Urbana-Champaign.

Sheen, H. L. J. 1987. *MV Herald of Free Enterprise* (Her Majesty's Stationery Report of Court No. 8074 Formal Investigation). London.

Transportation Safety Board of Canada. 1999. *Compressor bursting on the container ship 'Canmar Spirit':* Marine Investigation Report No. M99LOO11.

U.K. P&I Club. 1997. *Human error: Analyses of major claims. Principal causes within the five major risk categories insured by the UK club.* London: P&I Club.

U.K. P&I Club. 2002–2004. *Manning.* London: P&I Club, www.ukpandi.com/ukpandi/infopool.nsf/html/lp_init_lpstats.

U.S. Coast Guard. 1995. *Prevention through people.* Washington, DC: Department of Transportation, Quality Action Team.

U.S. Coast Guard. 2006. *U.S. Coast Guard Captain of the Port Long Island Sound waterways suitability report for the proposed broadwater liquefied natural gas facility.* U.S. Department of Homeland Security, U.S. Coast Guard, Report released Sept 21, http://www.uscg.mil/d1/units/seclis/broadwater/wsrrpt/WSR%20Master%20Final.pdf.

Vicente, K. 2004. *The human factor: Revolutionizing the way people live with technology.* New York: Taylor & Francis.

Walraven, P. L. 1967. Future needs in maritime operations. *Ergonomics* 10(5): 607–9.

Wertheim, A. H. 1998. Working in a moving environment. *Ergonomics* 41(12): 1845–58.

Westrum, R. 1992. Cultures with requisite imaginations. In *Verification and validation of complex systems: Human factors issues,* ed. J. Wise, D. Hopkin, and P. Stager, 401–16. New York: Springer-Verlag.

Glossary

Accident: Unintended *event*, including system (human, organizational, or equipment) *failures* and/or other mishaps, the consequences or potential consequences of which are not negligible from the point of view of maritime pollution prevention or safety. In this regard the IMO defines *accidents* (or maritime casualties), when this results "in death, serious injury, damage and/or loss of a vessel, and/or major pollution."

Active error: An error that occurs at the frontline level of operations (by an individual or group) and whose effects are felt almost immediately.

Anthropometry: The study of human body measurements that assists in understanding human physical variations and aids in workplace design to ensure appropriate fit between various elements of the system.

Bosun: Crew position on board a ship. It is the highest ranking deck rating who has immediate charge of all deck ratings and who in turn comes under the direct orders of the master and/or deck officers.

Bridge: Navigating section of the vessel where the wheelhouse and chartroom are located.

Classification society: An independent organization that certifies that a ship has been built and maintained according to the organization's rules for that type of ship. A ship that receives its certification is referred to as being "in-class." It is not compulsory that a vessel be built according to the rules of any classification society; but in practice, the difficulty in securing satisfactory insurance rates for an "unclassed" vessel makes it a commercial obligation.

Crew: Refers to the whole ship's complement such as masters, officers, and ratings.

Fatigue: A blanket term that covers internal states and performance decrements usually associated with either a need for sleep or tasks/environments that are mentally/physically demanding or insufficiently stimulating.

Flag state: The flag under which the ship is registered. The flag state is responsible to ensure that vessels registered under its flag meet IMO, ILO, and other international and national requirements.

Human error: An inappropriate or undesirable human decision or behavior that leads to undesirable outcomes or has significant potential for such an outcome. Accumulation of errors may result in accidents.

Human factors: Defined by the International Ergonomics Association as the scientific discipline concerned with the understanding of the interactions among humans and other elements of a system. The profession that applies theory, principles, data, and methods to design and operation in order to optimize human well-being and overall system performance. Sometimes used synonymously with ergonomics, but ergonomics is actually a subset of human factors.

Human factors research: The scientific acquisition of information about human capabilities and limitations related to equipment, facilities, procedures, jobs, organizations, environments, training, staffing, errors, situational awareness, workload, personnel management, people, and other performance implications in which the human is a component in meeting safety and capability objectives.

Human–machine interface: Or Man–Machine Interface (MMI). Concerned with the area of the human and the area of the machine that interact during a given task. The aim is to design a comfortable, stress- and hazard-free environment compatible with effective performance. The term is essentially equivalent to Human–Computer Interaction (HCI), except that it is used more often to refer to hardware, whereas HCI is used most often to refer to software.

ILO: International Labor Organization, a specialized agency of the United Nations involved over the years in appraising and seeking to improve and regulate labor conditions. Involved in such maritime areas as crew accommodation, accident prevention, medical examination and medical care, food and catering, and officer competency.

IMO: The International Maritime Organization, a specialized agency of the United Nations responsible for regulatory measures aimed to improve the safety of international shipping and prevention of marine pollution from ships.

Incident: Often used to describe *events* that are, in effect, minor accidents, that is, that are distinguished from accidents only in terms of being less severe. Note, however, this is an arbitrary distinction with little basis in normal usage. The IMO defines incidents as "an occurrence or event being caused by, or in connection with, the operation of a ship by which the ship or any person is imperilled, or as a result of which serious damage to the ship or structure or the environment might be caused."

ISM: International Safety Management code (ISM Code; Chapter IX of SOLAS).

ISO: International Standards Organization, body responsible for industrial standardization.

Job aids: The use of procedures, signs, and other written material to assist in ensuring the work process is remembered.

Latent error: Errors in the design, organization, training, or maintenance that lead to operator errors and whose effects typically lie dormant in the system for lengthy periods of time.

Maritime safety: The establishment of operational systems and processes that minimize the likelihood of errors and maximize the likelihood of intercepting them when they occur to ensure maritime safety.

MSC: Maritime Safety Committee, a major committee within the International Maritime Organization.

P&I Clubs: Protection and Indemnity Association, which is formed by ship owners to provide liability indemnification protection from various liabilities to which they are exposed in the course of their business. It spreads the liability costs of each member by requiring contribution by all members in the event of a loss.

Near miss: A potential significant *event* that could have occurred as the consequence of a sequence of actual occurrences but did not occur owing to the system conditions prevailing at the time. Near misses are considered similar to incidents; however, the outcome is total recovery with no damage or injury sustained.

Open registries: A term used in place of "flags of convenience" to denote registry in a country that offers favorable tax, regulatory, and other incentives to ship owners from other nations. They also allow crewing of ships with crew nationalities other than that of the flag state.

Performance-shaping factors: Factors that may influence human behavior sometimes determining the likelihood of error.

Port side: The left-hand side of a ship facing forward. The port side of a ship during darkness is indicated by a red light.

Port state control: The inspection of foreign ships in national ports for the purpose of verifying that the condition of a ship and its equipment is compliant with international conventions. If a substantial number of deficiencies are found, the ship may be detained until the necessary repairs have been carried out to the satisfaction of the port state control authority.

Ratings: Crew positions on board other than officers. Includes such positions as Able Seamen (AB) and leading Seamen (LS).

Ro-ro: Roll-on/roll-off vessels. These vessels are designed for cargo that can self-load on board. Cargo generally drives in and out of decks via ramps, rather than being lifted through hatches.

Seaworthiness: The sufficiency of a vessel to carry out its intended voyage safely. Any sort of disrepair to the vessel, such design deficiencies, overloading, untrained officers, lack of maintenance, may constitute a vessel being unseaworthy.

Ship management: The technical administration of a ship, including services like technical operation, maintenance, repair, crewing, and insurance.

Sociotechnical system: A systematic approach for viewing human factors; indicates how various elements interact to influence system performance. These elements may be both human and technology.

SOLAS: International Convention for the Safety of Life at Sea (IMO).

Starboard side: The right-hand side of a ship when facing forward. The starboard side of a ship during darkness is indicated by a green light.

STCW: International Convention on Standards of Training, Certification and Watchkeeping for Seafarers, 1978.

Index

Vicente, K.
  systematic approach 19
Vigilance 46
Visibility
  lighting 97
Vision 34–36
  foveal vision 34
  night vision 34
  parafoveal field 34, 36
  peripheral field 34
Visual
  attention 34
  comfort 97
  performance 96

W

Walk-through evaluations 162
Warnings 118–120, 151–152
  crew decisions 120
  use of pictorial information 119
  use of symbols 119
Watch schedules
  Human factors research 5

Watchkeeping
  fatigue 14
  single-person 125
Westrum, R.
  safety culture 138
Whole Body Vibrations 94
Woods, D.D. 47
Work environment 12, 89
Work overload 53
Work-related musculoskeletal disorders 67
  back injuries 67
  repetitive strain injuries 67
Work rest scheduling
  fatigue 6
Working memory 44
Workplace hazards 142
Workstation design 68–69
  adjustability 68
  clearance 68
  component arrangement 69
  reach 68
  seating 69
  visibility 69

Milton Keynes UK
Ingram Content Group UK Ltd.
UKHW020313111024
449327UK00040B/650